Praise for

The Interpretation
of Cats

"Fascinating. A must for every cat owner."

—Philippa Perry, author of
The Book You Want Everyone You Love to Read

"The internationally renowned veterinarian and animal psychologist Claude Béata has given cat lovers the perfect guide to their feline companions. Drawing on many years of experience and research into the behavior of these adorable and enigmatic creatures, he shows how they interact with the humans with whom they share their lives. If you want to understand the needs of cats, you can do no better than read this wise, witty, and absorbing book."

—John Gray, author of *Feline Philosophy*

"It is often said that there are two means of refuge from life—music and cats—and I'd like to add reading this book to this soul-healing prescription."

—Theresa Cheung, author of *Psychic Cats*

The Interpretation of Cats

Understanding the Psychology of Our Feline Companions

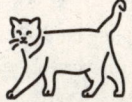

Dr. Claude Béata

Translated by David Watson

SCRIBNER

New York Amsterdam/Antwerp London
Toronto Sydney/Melbourne New Delhi

Scribner
An Imprint of Simon & Schuster, LLC
1230 Avenue of the Americas
New York, NY 10020

First Scribner paperback edition November 2025

SCRIBNER and design are trademarks of Simon & Schuster, LLC

Simon & Schuster strongly believes in freedom of expression and stands against censorship in all its forms. For more information, visit BooksBelong.com.

For information about special discounts for bulk purchases, please contact Simon & Schuster Special Sales at 1-866-506-1949 or business@simonandschuster.com.

The Simon & Schuster Speakers Bureau can bring authors to your live event. For more information or to book an event, contact the Simon & Schuster Speakers Bureau at 1-866-248-3049 or visit our website at www.simonspeakers.com.

Interior design by Kyle Kabel

Manufactured in the United States of America

1 3 5 7 9 10 8 6 4 2

Library of Congress Control Number: 2024943749

ISBN 978-1-6680-7065-9
ISBN 978-1-6680-7066-6 (pbk)
ISBN 978-1-6680-7067-3 (ebook)

Contents

Introduction

There she is. Crouched down on the floor. A black cat.

We are face to face. She is an impressive sight.

Anyone who has found themselves confronted by a feline that is about to pounce will know exactly what I am talking about.

Her ears are pinned back on her head, so flat they have almost disappeared.

She stares at me, and her intense gaze promises a combat without mercy. Her body is squat, and I sense the power in her muscles, tensed for attack, and I know I will have little chance to escape the sharp fangs and the tearing claws. I shift slightly to shake off the sense of unease that this menacing ball of flesh has instilled in me, but, like a warrior at the peak of her art, she does not take her eyes off me, and her imperceptible movement offers me no opening.

And yet, just five minutes earlier, I was close to being able to touch her; I even thought I might be able to stroke her. I could already feel the softness of her fur and the suppleness of her body beneath my hand. I had expected her to relax, our connection confirmed by a low purr, but an ever so slightly clumsy move on my part had broken the pact, and now we are back to square one. My status has changed: I am the enemy, someone to be suspicious of, whose every move will be interpreted as an attack and will unleash a retaliation.

I know she is scared. Me too.

And yet she weighs just six or seven pounds and I much more. But superior size and weight won't guarantee the outcome of the confrontation.

There we are, face to face, me a young vet, she a cat brought in for a routine checkup. Taking advantage of a moment of inattention, she has escaped from her cage and is now poised to defend herself. I am impressed by her determination. I crouch down and talk softly to her, endeavoring not to give her any cause to run off or to attack. I tell her how brave she is, how impressive. That I chose this profession to take care of her, to help her live a better life in our world, and to look after her well-being. She pricks up her ears a little, blinks her eyes; she seems to be saying that I have a way to go yet, that I have a lot to learn about how to communicate with her species, and with her in particular. I make my excuses, but they aren't good enough: I've lost her confidence, and it won't be that easy to win it back. It takes a whole quarter of an hour to get hold of her again without sustaining any injury and to learn my first lesson.

That was then, thirty-five years ago. I made a promise to that cat and to myself that I would get better at it. I don't think that journey is complete, but recently I had a strange dream: I was dressed like a student on graduation day—full gown and mortarboard—yet the panel of academics before me consisted purely of cats. I was familiar with quite a few of them. I recognized cats from my own life—Minou, Chiquita, my pal Al, Opium, Moustache, Flora. But also cats I had treated—Nougatine, Hannibal, Nougat. They called me up onto the stage and handed me my degree . . . the feline-language translator and president of the panel was none other than Prima, that cat from my first professional encounter that had made such an impression on me. She made a brief declaration: "We are the cats, lords of ancient legends and icons of social media. While we have often been praised for our qualities, even deified, we have also been martyred, nailed to the doors of barns, and cursed for imaginary transgressions. In all of this, I do not think that we have been understood." She then made a request to me—to write this book. "Can you help us? You owe us that much. Explain how we are both easy to understand and complex in the variety of our behaviors. Explain that, even though we are the cutest things imaginable when we are kittens, we deserve more than some fleeting fame on the internet. We have a rich, almost infinite repertoire of behaviors, and yet in that richness also lies our weakness. To you, who have cared for us, we give the mission of deciphering this craziness all around us and sometimes inside us, to explain how what we are can cause us psychological distress. And how, even though our brains are complex enough to allow us to adapt to almost anything, they are also fragile enough to sometimes make us 'mad.'"

Today, I hope to have fulfilled that task, and you have it in your hands: this book, which is dedicated to all my feline patients.

The Interpretation of Cats

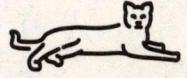

The Joker, or the Dual Nature of the Cat

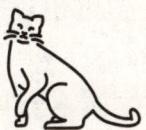

God created the cat so that man might have a tiger to stroke at home.

—*Victor Hugo*

Anyone who has seen their cat on the alert, or bringing home the prey it patiently hunted, or defending its territory against a dog ten times bigger than itself, will know that felines are perfectly adapted to fighting. Why have we deliberately chosen to live with such a lethal weapon? Because while recognizing cats' hunting prowess we also appreciate their capacity for emotional attachment and to express a preference, which makes our relationship with them so precious. That said, given that our shared life with cats is much more recent than ours with dogs, we might still feel that we are allowing a touch of wildness into our home.

Not So Sweet Nougat

At times one gets the feeling that the tiger is not far beneath the surface. For instance, ten years ago, when I first met a young European Shorthair kitten called Nougat, I could never quite forget that there was a big cat lurking inside him. When my client Angèle first called me about her four-month-old kitten, she mentioned that she was in a wheelchair and it was difficult for her to get around. We therefore set up a consultation at her house, which is always a risky undertaking when it comes to assessing a cat's behavior.

I had learned the hard way that house visits can be particularly tricky. When I was still in general practice working as a regular vet, a client had convinced me to come and vaccinate her cat at her home to avoid the struggles she faced every time she took him to the vet. "You'll see: at home he will be sweetness and light," she assured me. I didn't quite believe her, but seeing that she was quite emotional, I agreed to give it a go. When I got there, I put my finger to the bell and, even before I could alert her to my presence, I could hear the cat hissing inside. As my client let me into her apartment, she said apologetically: "I don't know how he knew you were there, but he has fled to the top of the cupboard." And up there, with the advantage of height, and oblivious to the fact that we meant him no harm but just wanted to look after him, he was ready to defend himself to the hilt, at the cost of our hands and faces. We had to give up and arrange an appointment at the clinic instead.

Based on this previous experience, I shared my concern with Nougat's owner, but she assured me that he wouldn't disappear. When I arrived, Angèle was accompanied by Agnès, a neighbor who helped her out around the house: she had known Nougat since he had first arrived and summed him up in a word: "He is a devil!"

Barely had I sat down at a table with them to learn the short history of this cat and the main symptoms he presented when he jumped onto my lap and from thence to the table. From there he leaped on top of the TV (quite a large one) and tipped over a small pot containing a succulent. "It's like this all the time," said Angèle with a sigh. "I've never met such a clumsy cat."

These days, I treat this kind of behavior as a major element in my semiological analysis (gathering together behavioral signs that I interpret as symptoms) even though it is not officially a criterion in the diagnosis of hypersensitivity–hyperactivity syndrome (HSHA). We know how skillful cats are when they leap—the way they can sometimes land in the middle of a row of knickknacks on a mantelpiece without knocking anything over. But when we see a cat take so little care in the way it lands that it ends up breaking things, this points to a lack of self-control. Today we are more familiar with the prevalence of HSHA syndrome in the canine species: dogs have an automatic, unconscious capacity to coordinate and control essential movements having to do with locomotion and bite.[1] Cats have the same ability to control not only biting and locomotion but also scratching.

It is rare for a cat to be simply clumsy. When this is flagged, we check two particular points: the type of clumsiness and how dangerous it is (see box).

How to Understand Clumsiness in a Cat

Is it clumsiness or communication? Many cats tip over their empty bowl at mealtimes while retaining perfect mastery of their movements: in this case, it is simply a message, a reminder of what time it is and the cat's way of requesting food. It has no pathological significance.

Has the cat's clumsiness placed it in any danger? In the same way that hyperactive dogs are more prone to accidents in the home, HSHA cats also tend to pay a high price. "Parachute" cats who fall from balconies too often for it to be by chance, cats who swallow inedible objects out of greed and lack of due caution: we see many such cases in general practice and surgery, and these days most vets alert owners to the abnormal nature of such behavior and the options for care.

Things hadn't quite gotten to that stage with Nougat, now watching me from his perch on top of the TV. I moved a pen across the table and he was with me in a flash. Angèle had warned me: "Watch out: when he plays, he is like a tiger. . . ." And here he was, a wild beast indeed. I teased Nougat by hiding my hand under the table and scratching the tabletop from below, briefly flashing my fingers at him. For a cat, this reproduces the classic behavior of prey that hides away but at some point emerges from its burrow. Nougat pounced on my hand, fast as lightning, teeth and claws bared. Every contact with him resulted in minor injuries, which was not normal. When kittens play, and if they have developed properly, they are capable of controlling their mouth and claws. They play-act predation—it's part of their education—but it's a game and should not cause harm. Nougat, however, used his claws and teeth, and both Agnès and Angèle confirmed that they no longer played with him to avoid getting hurt. And because no one played with him, Nougat had to provide his own stimulus. The happy mess of this apartment was a paradise for a cat: there were hiding places everywhere and many ways to take advantage of them.

Nougat displayed behavior that was weird, to say the least: he jumped inside an open box and hid himself (so far, so normal—lots of cats like to do that) before leaping out again and attacking a completely immobile piece of curling ribbon. Trapping it between his paws, he shredded it, then ran off, skidding down the hallway, until we heard the sound of an object being knocked over. Then, no sooner had he gone than he was back and once more on my lap. I tried to stroke him slowly and softly, but the mere touch of my hand set off a reaction: Nougat grabbed it with his rear legs, claws out, and bit it unceremoniously. Yet there was nothing in his attitude that hinted at aggression. The whole thing was doubtless just a game to him, though once again it displayed a total lack of control. To verify this, I acted like a mother cat with her kitten and gave him a few gentle taps on the nose with my fingers. Anyone who has observed mother cats raising their offspring will know that they do so with patience, firmness, and consistency to inculcate control of the teeth and claws. This can take different forms.

A few years ago, I did a TV program on the development of babies, dogs, and cats, in which we studied a Nebelung cat,* Letti, and the way she behaved. A camera filmed her continuously over a few days, and we were able to observe that she spent a lot of time controlling her kittens. We never saw her be too tough on them. When a kitten passed over her without showing enough respect, Letti grabbed it between her paws and immobilized it for a few seconds before letting it go again. The kittens quickly learned that they had to lie still and wait until the friendly maternal taps or pressure ceased. But Nougat did not react at all in this way: whenever I reached out my hand to give him little flicks with my fingers, he retaliated with a strong swipe of his paw and, within a few seconds, drew blood. Yet even if it looked like an act of aggression, the sequence of events was more like play or an uncontrolled response.

A Matter of Self-Control

"You see, there's nothing we can do," lamented Angèle's friend Agnès. "He jumps on us, bites us, and even when we try to

---

* A blue-gray cat, a bit like a Russian Blue, but long-haired.

play with him, he soon draws blood. Angèle can't cope with this in her wheelchair, with all her treatments." Agnès likewise complained about "constant attacks" by the kitten. I suggested an experiment to see to what extent Nougat was capable of change. I asked her to begin playing with him, and as soon as he bared his claws, to stop interacting with him completely, put her hands on her head, and "make like a tree"—that is, not move at all or even look at her attacker. Agnès went along with this: Nougat climbed onto her and bit her hands. At my signal, she became a tree and didn't bat an eyelid. The kitten was a bit taken aback, but cats have more resources than dogs in the face of such immobility, and Nougat found a way around it. He turned to Agnès's heels and nipped her quite hard. She reacted and moved again, which set off further reactions from the cat. So that ploy didn't work, and, remember, he was four or five pounds of pure tiger.

I recorded further symptoms and was later able to establish that Nougat ticked all the boxes of stage 2 hypersensitivity-hyperactivity syndrome. He was voracious to the point of vomiting and, typically, he was a thief. He slept very little and always seemed to be on the prowl. Nowadays we know how to take care of such cats, and our two-pronged treatment—behavioral and medical—yields very good results, allowing a cat to be kept at home and reintegrated into family life.

In those days, when TVs were still chunky enough to act as landing strips and launchpads for kittens, I was hesitant about prescribing the psychotropic drug suitable for a four-month-old. It is a fault in the regulation of certain neurotransmitters, particularly serotonin, that is at the root of this developmental problem, and one of our treatments of choice is fluoxetine (Prozac). Unfortunately, this product tends to have a bad reputation, and everyone who has taken this antidepressant, or who knows someone who has, is familiar with its mixed results. Veterinarians use it as a medicine of control, and it has saved the lives of thousands of dogs and cats by helping them—always as a complement to behavioral therapy—to recover their self-control mechanisms. Back when I met Nougat, the theory was that we should wait until the end of an animal's maturation before using such a product, thus no earlier than six or eight months. Nougat was given another treatment, which did not control him enough, and Angèle and Agnès could no longer tolerate all the bites and scratches, which could have had disastrous medical consequences. A few weeks later, I found out that Nougat had been given to a friend with a house in the country. I understood the reasons for this decision and did not blame them. But one couldn't hold out much hope for this hyperactive cat and his new outdoor life: the chances of survival were not that great when there were no self-control mechanisms in place.

Even though my encounter with Nougat took place a decade ago, it has remained lodged in my mind as a cautionary tale, and after discussing the matter with fellow psychiatrists at a later date, we decided that the age guidance for fluoxetine was counterproductive. Nowadays, if the symptoms require it, I prescribe fluoxetine from the age of three or four months in order to save the life of a kitten.

This lack of control was not Nougat's fault: we now know that the roots of illness are a mixture of genetic vulnerability and developmental circumstances, and that the presence of a mother who is herself well-balanced is a crucial element in the formation of self-control mechanisms. Let us not forget that, under the surface, a domestic cat is still potentially a wild animal, and it is important to realize this and understand the causes of illness and the consequences. Cats are not small dogs; their behavior is different, and the story of Nougat reminds us how any imbalance can bring out the predator within.

A Little History

Twenty thousand years after the first dogs started living with humans, another carnivore came to share their everyday life. Where dogs and humans had a close-knit social bond and a common interest, this new addition was taken on primarily as a killer.

We said to cats: you can come and live with us, eat our leftovers, drink milk from our cows, enjoy the warmth of our fires, on the condition that you get rid of the mice and rats who raid the grain from our harvests. Cats only came to live with us when we settled down to become agricultural societies. Their presence was the product of a radical change in the human lifestyle; we learned to accommodate the presence of felines despite mutual distrust.

Can you imagine what it must have been like for our distant ancestors, in Asia or Africa, or even in Europe, at the time of the cave paintings at Lascaux and Chauvet? Whether saber-toothed tigers—they disappeared much later (10,000 years ago) than the original estimates (500,000 years ago)— or cave lions, which dwelt in these famous caves, cats would have immediately conjured an image of cunning and mortal danger. They acted alone, often in the shadows, and with their fangs and claws they spelled almost certain death to their chosen victims. This atavistic fear no doubt still lurks deep in the human imagination, and when Tiddles starts acting like a tiger or a lion, he reawakens in us that same terror of the prey.

The first felines appeared 12 to 13 million years ago, and the thirty-seven members of the Felidae family still have very similar characteristics. Even the best specialists can get it wrong when trying to distinguish a lion's skull from that of a tiger. There are three recognized genera. The *Panthera* all like to roar. As everyone knows, only cheetahs have claws that don't retract and they are the sole members of the genus *Acinonyx*. As for all the other "small" cats, they are to be found in the genus *Felis*.

Cats are unique. Nowadays, they are one of the animals most sought after as a pet, but, apart from pedigree cats, which make up a very small percentage of the cat population, the term "domesticated" is not appropriate. Indeed, for it to be applied correctly, the species must depend on humans for reproduction, breeding, and all its needs. This domestication changes the morphology of the species, taking it away from its wild roots. Even today, despite the best efforts of many protectors and owners, cat reproduction still evades human control. I believe we are taking a wrong turn by introducing mass sterilization for all family cats. We risk being left only with pedigree or rescue cats.

Hypertypes

Like many of my colleagues today, I see the damage created by absurd breeding practices that lead to the existence of hypertypes, in which traits specific to pedigree cats are accentuated to an extreme degree. Even if the intention is to improve the cat species, I am no fan of the idea of leaving the future of the species in the hands of breeders. There are cat shows, for example, where higher marks go to Persian cats with concave faces—cats whose noses are set deeper than their eyes. They have more breathing difficulties, and their quality of life is not good. We vets are the guardians of animal welfare, but often our voices go unheard in the breeding clubs, and our warnings are ignored.

For a few years my family and I shared our lives with a Sphynx cat called Galinette. We loved her; she was unique, mischievous, affectionate, and we mourned her greatly when she'd gone. But for me she wasn't a cat: although she had access to the outdoors, for her leaving the house was purgatory. Her pretty blue eyes couldn't stand the sun, and as for her skin, the slightest contact with plants gave her pruritus, and she would break out in a rash. Of her own accord, she greatly restricted her excursions.

It is harsh of me to say that she wasn't a cat. For example, she was a great predator, though in her own particular way. I amused generations of vets by filming her playing on hunt simulators on the iPad: she could concentrate on it for more than a quarter of an hour. I think one day she even amassed more than 2,000 points on *Games for Cats!*

I take such exception to this excessive selection (and these days most vets across the world think along the same lines)[2] because it causes suffering. Galinette suffered from a very young age. We adopted her because she had feline calicivirus (a respiratory virus) and had become unsellable for her breeder. This had nothing to do with her breeding. She didn't live very long (four years) and she died of the equivalent of Charcot-Marie-Tooth disease, a degeneration of the neuromuscular plaque, which was diagnosed by a laboratory in San Diego, California, and which may have been a consequence of her selection. Her daily discomfort was directly linked to her particularity: her lack of fur made her skin very fragile, and the fatty seborrhea that often occurs with the absence of hair made her the only cat in the family that stained all the fabrics on which she lay down. In her favorite spots, the stains were impossible to remove. In spite of that—and sometimes because of her very frailty—we had a close bond with her.

I think I can say that she was happy: to us she seemed full of joy, as cuddly as we could wish. Though Galinette was an extraordinary character, her breed is an assault on the dignity of cats. Currently, several countries are legislating to ban certain breeds of cats (and dogs), when the selection of a hypertype affects their well-being. It seems a shame to me that we have to turn to the law: it suggests reasoned argument was not enough. It also runs the risk of creating a black market where the animals will be traded with even less regard for their well-being.

In Belgium in February 2021, the Walloon Council for Animal Welfare asked for the immediate banning of four breeds: the Scottish Fold, with its folded ears, which has many followers; the tailless Manx cat; the Munchkin with very short legs; and the Twisty or Kangaroo cat, with its atrophied or twisted limbs. The council also required the creation of a special commission for four other breeds: the Persian, the Exotic Shorthair, the Sphynx, and the Devon Rex. If such an organization had existed before and had been created in France, an unlikely blue-eyed and light-skinned cat would not have come into our lives, and we would have gladly given up those few years of affectionate companionship to avoid so much suffering.

I say all this to emphasize how entrusting the future of the feline species to breeders alone would not be sensible. But I have no doubt that we can all work together to improve the well-being of all pedigree cats by significantly limiting the number of hypertypes.

Rescue Cats

When it comes to rescue cats, I believe we should adopt them, of course, but it is not sacrilegious to say that there is a greater risk of behavioral problems with them. Some of them are abandoned because of problems with cleanliness or aggression (those two things alone account for 80 percent of medical consultations relating to cat behavioral issues). Disorders are not consistently managed in cat shelters: often they do not show up at all, or to only a very limited degree, under these very different conditions, and veterinary or volunteer staff are not trained in diagnosis or treatment, whether biological or behavioral.

Even when cats without problems arrive at a shelter, being in such a large community of other cats can create new issues. A cat needs to control its territory and have separate spaces, and this is often impossible to achieve at a shelter despite the best efforts of the charity workers and volunteers.

If you visit a cat shelter, you will see colonies of cats sharing a space. The people in charge say there are very few confrontations between cats, and whenever I have spent some time at one, this has seemed to be the case.

On the other hand, there are sometimes clear signs of depression among the feline inmates: when you visit these places, you will mainly find calm animals. With a more experienced eye you may notice cats with tangled, matted fur, a sign that they have been stinting on their grooming. It's an indication of what experimental psychology calls *learned helplessness*. This phenomenon was described in the mid-1960s by Martin Seligman and Steven Maier in dogs following controversial experiments that won't be repeated.[3] Their theory posited that learned helplessness leads an animal to lose the sense of a connection between how it acts and the outcome of that action, the ability to have an awareness about that, and a behavioral response. Their experiment, conducted on dogs and reproduced on other animals, might have served as a demonstration of the existence of autonomous thought and the possibility of depression in animals, but it went against the orthodoxy of the time. When an animal finds itself in a situation in which its actions no longer affect its environment, and it can form an imaginary picture of its situation, then it displays behaviors that don't make any sense. Lack of grooming fits in, as does massive behavioral inhibition. This suggests the possibility of a psychopathology, and we can see clear symptoms of a depressive state. The work of Seligman and Maier has been much used in human psychiatry as well to study depression.

So if you adopt a cat from a cat shelter, because its personality might have been affected and because of the time it has spent at the shelter, you run the risk of inviting depression into your home. One has to be aware the animal may have suffered major psychological trauma. Obviously, some cats have a natural resilience that will enable them to find their balance, but how many will never be able to trust their new owner, never be able to get over their pathological inhibition?

Sensitivity and Inhibition

This is the second aspect of a cat's nature. As we have seen from how their history has played out, cats are predators, but they are also prey, and that predisposes them to two types of pathological process: hypersensitivity and inhibition. We will be revisiting these over the course of this book as they are key to understanding a great many of the problems in cats.

Behavioral inhibition is one of the three ways of reacting to frightening or unpleasant stimuli. It is known as the 3F rule: *fight, flight, or freeze*. These three behavioral responses are not abnormal in themselves; in many situations they may guarantee survival. Sometimes, though, they become the symptoms of a behavioral condition. The distinction between normal and pathological is often complicated, perhaps even more so in my field. We have established three factors that indicate pathology: absence of adaptability, absence of spontaneous reversibility, and suffering.

Indeed, this is the very definition of a depressive state: a state of inhibition that is not reversible in a natural way, that prevents the individual from adapting optimally to their environment and causes them daily suffering. It's the fate of many cats that are locked up. That isn't a reason not to adopt them; it might in fact be an extra incentive to do so, if it is done consciously.

Houdini, the Cat Who Never Gave Up

Some cats overcome their fate, and I can't talk about rescue cats without mentioning Houdini. A few years ago, I visited a shelter on the outskirts of Paris, an example of how well run a place like that can be under the supervision of an extraordinarily devoted team. Every dog cage had a label with the animal's history and behavioral characteristics marked on it. We went to the cat house, where I was astonished to see there was a section for cats suffering from serious and contagious viral conditions. I asked why this was, and a manager replied: "Oh, they are quite easy to place. We have a particular 'clientele' who say, 'Give me the cat that no one wants; I live in an apartment, I don't have any other cats, so he can be sick, contagious, whatever. I'll make sure he's taken care of and give him the best possible life.' And so what might have been a real problem becomes a surefire way of guaranteeing a placement."

I'd barely overcome my surprise when a volunteer said: "Be careful! Houdini is behind that door! If you approach quietly and look through the window in the door, you might see him getting ready to make a bolt for it." On tiptoes, phone in hand to capture the moment, I approached and was able to take a picture of the cat scoping out his potential escape route.

Most workers at the shelter had given up on him, but a few had hung in there. Houdini had escaped from his caregivers on countless occasions: that was the constant fear of the young recruits, and became something of a comedic initiation ceremony set up by the older hands. As soon as the cat heard someone approaching, he would lurk in a blind spot; the door would only have to open a crack and he would be outside in a flash. He was cunning, so he would never lurk in the same place twice. I could even imagine him on hind legs, his back flat to the wall, slim as a cigarette paper, ready to slip out through the narrowest gap.

He, of course, wasn't depressive, but it's too much to expect most cats to have the determination of Papillon or of Captain Virgil Hilts, "the Cooler King," played so brilliantly by Steve McQueen in *The Great Escape*. Houdini never gave up—he is a testament to the fact that the worst is never a done deal—but you need exceptional amounts of resistance and resilience, and never-ending hope, to be able to tolerate incarceration without lapsing into resignation. I didn't hear about him after that, but I imagine him still leaping at every opportunity for that elusive means of escape.

Domesticated? Never!

I wouldn't want us only to be able to acquire cats from breeders or cat shelters. To forbid responsible individuals to allow their house cat, which is civilized and used to other animals, to reproduce would be a significant attack on freedom as well as scientifically nonsensical.

Cats live with us, but they aren't completely domesticated.

Maybe that's part of the secret of their success: as Victor Hugo's aphorism at the head of this chapter puts it, inviting a cat into your home involves accepting a wild beast. You are welcoming the "other," in all its familiarity and its strangeness. As the French philosopher Baptiste Morizot reminds us: "When we open our eyes, what we see is both an alien and a relative."[4] That's the case with our domestic felines. Sometimes they are predictable, friendly, and cute, then suddenly their behavior can seem completely mystifying.

In the face of such baffling behavior, which can seem like an uncrackable strongbox with five locks, I will offer you several keys over the course of the following chapters, and I hope they will allow you to acquire a better understanding of cats in general, and of those you encounter daily.

The first key, and probably the most important one, which we will see has significant consequences, is to attempt to understand the cat's dual nature as both prey and predator. Cats are the champions of "being two things at once." In fact, it is quite rare that a single species takes the paradox of excelling in each aspect of its nature to such an extreme: being an efficient and fearsome hunter while in the blink of an eye developing strategies of avoidance and self-protection from a presumed predator or some other danger.

I filmed a scene in my garden that taught me a lot about this. My teachers were our young cat Chiquita (without doubt one of my best instructors) and a dwarf lop-eared rabbit called Avoine who derived a lot of enjoyment from our little square of greenery. Chiquita, who was barely four months old, had spotted Avoine in the garden and was creeping forward on her belly, like a lioness on the savannah advancing downwind toward an antelope. The rabbit, who already had several cats under her belt, and who, while nominally a dwarf, nonetheless weighed three or four times more than the young cat, saw her coming out of the corner of her eye. Just as Chiquita gathered herself, ready to pounce, Avoine suddenly pinned her down, and in the blink of an eye the tables had been turned, and the cat was forced to flee from this unforeseen threat. For her whole life up to that point, Chiquita had been very well-balanced, so this wasn't such a terrible experience for her, but it did illustrate that ever-possible shift from one pole of her life to the other—being a top-notch hunter and yet of a size that exposed her to being hunted herself. In this, cats are like secret agents: their license to kill implies that they might themselves be killed.

This everyday scene illustrates fundamental truths about the profound nature of cats. They each possess the complete behavioral kit of the predator but also the adaptive needs of the prey. That is what makes them complex and unique. It's a bit like a lottery. Consider that the predator has twenty to twenty-five primordial behaviors and the prey has roughly the same number, but of a different kind. Consider also that each animal has one of the ten or so main personality types, drawn at random in the genetic game of chance (which have less to do with the species, and more with the lineage and the individual). This combination of personality and the five major forms of behavior that make up what we might call the dominant behavioral phenotype of this animal—that is, its expression as an individual—represents a lottery draw of five of the forty-nine (or fifty) behaviors of prey and predator, along with the five-pronged star of personality, which makes for over 20 million possible variations.

Each cat is unique, as anyone who has lived with several cats will know. Chiquita, who taught me a lot—as much about empathy as about the predator–prey duality of the feline character—had three kittens: ginger Ron, tiger-striped

Harry, and tortoiseshell Hermione. They were as different as they could be. The daughter of a well-balanced cat, sister of two equally serene, even bold brothers, Hermione has always been rather fearful. Living with us and her mother, she has faced no alarming situations. Nevertheless, we have always had the feeling that she felt threatened by some great danger. Chiquita was a protective mother, maybe even a little overbearing. We sometimes feel that, when kittens maintain contact with their mother, it is harder for their development to be completed properly, and the animal ends up being less mature and not so independent. In any case, these three kittens and their mother (we never knew the father) were an example of the diverse range of feline behavior and of the relative independence of a cat's personality from its genetic family.

While each cat is unique, they are all defined by the tension between these two poles of their feline nature. When the processes inherent in the status of prey become exaggerated in a cat, this can give rise to many problems, but the predator side too can cause damage.

We have already seen Nougat and the consequences of his uncontrolled play: what was just a game to him turned out to be unpleasant, harmful, even dangerous for his owner. Play for a cat is always an apprenticeship for adult life or a repetition of primordial scenes. When a cat plays at being a predator, it mimics all the moves but—and this is the whole point of play—never forgets that it is not for real, so has no need to use the full force of its claws or fangs.

The predatory side of a cat's nature also expresses itself in abnormal fashion in two other instances: in an environment lacking even minimal stimuli; and where there are mood problems. This shows us that the same symptom, abnormal predation, can arise from different causes—whether a developmental problem such as hyperactivity, unfavorable environmental conditions, or problems of mood—and it is crucial to treat not just the symptom, but the whole individual.

The Desert of the Tartars

The simplest, and most common, instance is when an environment lacks even basic kinds of stimulus. Indulging in predatory activity, whether with real prey or with a lure, is a major element in a cat's well-being and quality of life. Abnormal symptoms will be even more pronounced the more the cat's environment differs from the one in which it initially developed.

Lucifer was a pretty black cat that Huguette was given by her grandchildren, who knew how sad she was when her old cat, Minou, died. And because they wanted to do the right thing, they got Lucifer from a cat shelter. He came from a litter that had been rescued, after a fortnight of patient work, from where they were hiding beneath a school playground.

Although Huguette was sad after losing Minou a few months earlier, she didn't really want a new feline companion: her life now was cloistered and lacking in stimulus, and she didn't want to impose this on a kitten. Huguette spent her days engaged in small manual tasks. She sewed, did embroidery, and thus spent much of her time doing needlework; she also wrote and kept her accounts up to date. Lucifer would jump onto the table, crouch, and then attack Huguette's hands as she used a needle or a pen. At first Huguette found this amusing. She thought it was just play, which was indeed the case, but before long she was being injured by these attacks and could no longer deal with it. As soon as she started to sanction Lucifer, giving him a few taps, the situation escalated, and his aggression became more harmful. She therefore brought him in for a consultation.

Lucifer was living in an environment that wasn't providing him with the minimum that was necessary for his equilibrium as a predator. He had to exercise his essential predatory nature at the expense of Huguette's exposed hands and ankles. All owners of cats that behave in this way tell the same story. They know the exact spot where the cat will crouch and get ready to spring on them and attack them. The first time it will take them by surprise. Subsequently, they will be less and less taken aback to find the cat behind the chest of drawers in the hallway or behind some other piece of furniture. When they walk by, their little tiger will pounce on their heels, seizing them between their incisors, sometimes even chewing them with their back teeth.

It was the same for Huguette: no sooner had she begun sewing or embroidering, or even writing, than Lucifer leaped onto her and bit her, sometimes painfully. Because he was in an environment where there were no options for exercising his hunting instincts, he redirected them at the only available target: Huguette. Some researchers have made films of women walking and shown how much they can resemble a bird hopping, especially if they are wearing heels. Granted, that seems a little far-fetched, but it's quite easy to understand how movement, any movement, in an environment without stimulus, can be an effective trigger for predatory responses in a cat. So these attacks are a direct consequence of a cat being cloistered in an environment devoid of stimulus. This used to be referred to as "cat anxiety in a closed space," which highlights the fact that the root of the problem lies in going from an open environment, in which the cat can catch prey and lurk, to a closed one in which hunting is not possible.

Indoors or Outdoors? A Dangerous Received Idea

We should pause here to make one thing clear. We are not at all saying that a cat can't be well-balanced if it lives indoors. All you need to do is have cat toys and organize hunting games. It is even more important to check that any cat that is going to stay indoors has started living its life this way. That will greatly facilitate their adaptation. It is obvious that a cat that is used to hunting natural prey outdoors will have difficulty adapting to being indoors all the time.

A student on our degree course undertook an interesting topic for her dissertation.[5] We wanted to verify something that seemed a matter of common sense and expressed by many educators and vets: how access to the outside, the possibility of leading a freer life, reduced the prevalence of behavioral issues in cats. We had our doubts about this, but without evidence to back it up it was difficult to discuss the matter properly. The study was very broad: it was based on more than 350 cats from nine veterinary practices, and it demonstrated that, in fact, contrary to what had been assumed, there were just as many behavioral issues among cats with access to the outside as among those without it.

Typically, those working in feline behavioral medicine hear two main complaints by clients regarding their cats: uncleanliness and aggression. The prevalence of such issues was found statistically to be no different for cats living outdoors, for those who could go outside whenever they liked, or for those with no access to the outside. It is quite common for our domestic cats to sit in front of a tap and wait until their human gives them access to running water. These days, the introduction of water fountains for cats covers this need. Nearly fifteen years ago, this request for access to running water was more frequent in confined cats than in those who had access to the outdoors and who could satisfy their need for clear water.

On these two major issues—aggression and uncleanliness—the situation was quite comparable. If there is a difference, it may have to do with the owners who choose to let their cats go out: they found it much worse than owners of "locked-up" cats, for example, to have to clear up urine or feces indoors when the cat could have done its business outside.

A Little Devil

Let's get back to Lucifer. Every day—especially, according to Huguette, in the late afternoon or early evening as daylight waned—he would start his predatory attacks on her hands. As Huguette was on anticoagulants, this posed a certain health risk. "I think he's a cute little cat," she told us. "I know he's just playing, but I don't understand why he wants to hurt me." Today, instead of calling it "cat anxiety in an enclosed space," psychiatric vets here in France use the term *aplouto-biotopathy*. That is to say that the cat's environment, which plays a big role in cat problems—as we will see in the next chapter—does not provide it with the minimum stimulus it needs to be well-balanced. A cat that is deprived of stimuli will invent them. It will therefore react to the types of stimulation that normally would not trigger anything, such as the movement of a pen or a needle, or even someone walking quietly in slippers. The owners of such cats cannot tolerate this and are often tempted to react by punishing the cat so that it begins to develop increasingly aggressive behavior.

Once the cat is sanctioned, the relationship with the human will deteriorate, the assaults becoming more and more violent, and their bond will gradually loosen: the harmony between them will disappear. When things come to this, as in the case of Lucifer and Huguette, it's time to call in the vet. If this is linked to unfavorable living conditions, then it leads quite quickly to a pathological state. At this point anxiety may be diagnosed, accompanied by displays of undesirable behavior such as uncleanliness or aggression, or behavioral inhibition and anxiety, or even depression, similar to what we saw in rescue cats when they didn't have enough stimulation.

Treating Anxiety

An employee forced to do a monotonous job every day or endure harassment may fall into a pathological state of anxiety or depression that won't simply go away once the toxic conditions are removed: they will need care. In the same way, cats displaying similar symptoms require some rearrangement of their environment that allows them to satisfy their needs, in addition to medical treatment, in order to restore their sensory homeostasis and equilibrium, helping them back to good health.

It is very important to remember this: look at Huguette. She sounds like many an elderly person faced with difficulties: "I knew it, I was too old. I shouldn't have taken on a new animal. I no longer have what it takes to give him what he needs." That's not true. It bears repeating: even in an indoor space, it is sufficient to provide a cat, for example, with the three-dimensional resources it needs, such as a scratching post and a cat tree to climb (see box). These tools aren't the answer to everything, but they can often improve a cat's quality of life.

Cat Tree

To work well, this device should be made up of several elements that will satisfy the basic needs of a cat. First, it should have a number of different levels. The varying heights allow a cat to choose the location of its zone of isolation and select one that is raised and enables it to feel protected. It should also provide a few hiding places, more or less closed boxes that give the cat a place to spy from—a favorite pastime for many felines. The "trunk" is usually wrapped in rope, which gives the cat something to scratch. And if the tree is placed next to a window and this provides an observation post, this simple piece of equipment offers a key to feline well-being . . . even if it is not enough in itself.

In every consultation, there are various lines of treatment. The first, very important step is to get a good grasp of the situation. The animal's companion, its owner, should understand what is taking place. I explained to Huguette that, in fact, this was not so different from the picture she herself had painted: that the environment offered to Lucifer undoubtedly needed to be enriched, and that this was eminently achievable without too much effort or expense.

The second, equally important, point is that an empathetic approach is needed, both with the owner and with the cat. Being regularly hunted by your cat and attacked by it is unpleasant and painful. Even if you realize that this has more to do with play than with aggression, you will still feel threatened. This is even more the case for elderly people, like Huguette, taking blood thinners, thereby exacerbating the risk of injury caused by her feline companion. The empathetic work with Huguette lay in acknowledging her disappointment and understanding her fears. It also involved making clear from the start that, even if Lucifer had "good" reasons for his behavior, there was no question that he would be allowed to get away with it. The difficulty often arises from the notion of punishment. For Huguette, and for many of our other clients, there is a belief that the animal should be punished in order to understand that it has behaved badly.

Disruption, Not Punishment

In feline behavioral medicine our first prescription is nearly always: stop the punishments. Not just physical punishment, but also raising the voice and making threats. Coercion is never part of the solution; it is only ever a source of aggravation. It's complicated because our society and our schooling, especially for people of a certain age, tends to have been based on punishment and repression. That is why for so long cats have had the reputation of never learning anything, because models of learning for dogs and horses, as they were for children, used to be based on punishment: a rap on the knuckles for schoolchildren, a crack of the whip for horses, a stick for dogs. These methods never work with cats: hurt them or scare them just once and you may destroy your relationship forever.

So you have to forbid without punishing—but how? Is there a way of preventing attacks without resorting to painful or frightening punishments? The solution lies in disruption. To interrupt an unwelcome action you could, for example, fire a jet of compressed air or water at the cat at the moment when it is about to spring: nothing dangerous or particularly scary there. That is why, if you come to the houses of some of my clients near my clinic, especially in the Toulon area, you will see grannies and grandpas walking around their apartments with water pistols strapped to their belts like John Wayne in a saloon. At the exact spot where the cat threatens to attack, from behind that chest of drawers where it lurks, at the precise moment when it appears, its intended victim draws their water pistol, plant mister, or keyboard cleaner and fires off a brief squirt. This reproduces the hissing sound a cat makes when it is being threatening, so it is easily understood by the animal without being painful or upsetting. In this way the risk of aggression against a person is reduced while at the same time, as I suggest to my clients, the attack is redirected to a lure, such as a feather or a plushie attached to the end of a toy fishing rod. This will spare the owner's calves or ankles while allowing the cat to behave as its nature dictates. In time, there will be no more injuries and so no further punishment. Fear will be reduced on both sides, harmony can be reestablished, and the cat can carry on living peaceably with its owner. Otherwise the cat runs the risk of being abandoned on the advice of children or doctors if it is considered to be a danger, especially to an older person.

The Importance of Medication

In the case of Lucifer and Huguette, I began by reducing impulsive aggression in order to treat the cat's anxiety. This involves the owners accepting the idea of medical treatment and our being able to give it. There is a whole range of treatments we can use these days, with different methods of administration, and some of these are more suitable for cats. Certain products can be administered without prescription, like pheromones, nutraceuticals (food sources with health benefits), and aromatherapy. Sometimes we have recourse to psychotropics, always on a veterinary prescription: some are designed for animals, and we obtain others from the human pharmacopoeia.

Vets can adapt their prescription according to the severity of the symptoms or according to how easy it is to manipulate the cat. There is always a solution. Sometimes we still encounter resistance. There may be a clash between the notion of a solitary, independent cat that cures itself and the idea of "giving it some drops" to prevent the excesses of its impulsive behavior. Such notions are changing, at a fast rate. Feline medicine has made huge progress in every field—from cardiology and dermatology to infectious diseases—and psychiatry is not standing still either.

For Lucifer I prescribed the psychotropic that works best for impulsiveness and I made sure Huguette knew how to administer it. She was positive about this: "He's fine with medicine, I can give him anything. . . . That's why I couldn't understand why he was so naughty sometimes, but now I understand a little better. . . . Which cat tree do you recommend?" I told her that this product would reduce her cat's impulsiveness and anxiety. It was also imperative to start putting in place the elements that would enrich his environment.

Enriching the Environment

I helped Huguette choose a cat tree that would fit in her apartment and that would provide all the desired functions mentioned above. I suggested a water pistol, which Huguette replaced with a plant spray bottle that she already had at home. Then we offered Lucifer various lures that could be attached to a toy fishing rod, from feathers to little stuffed mice. In this case you need to find out what really amuses the cat. You have to discover what will motivate it to chase after something and satisfy its fundamental need to hunt.

All this was put in place by Huguette. She wanted to keep her feline friend, despite his fearsome teeth and razor-sharp claws, who would come to sleep next to her on the sofa in the evening and who, for a brief but delicious interlude, would leap onto her lap and curl up in a ball, purring like an airplane engine for a few minutes before returning to his kitten games.

Two months later, no further wounds had been inflicted on Huguette by Lucifer. He had turned into a playful cat, full of joy and with lots of little hiding places around the house: he was mischievous, funny, and a source of great amusement to Huguette. They got along famously. Lucifer is living proof that psychotropics do not change personality but simply allow one—in this case—to control and tone down excessively impulsive behavior. Huguette respected her cat's feeding rhythm (at least six times a day), played with him, and helped him lead a well-balanced life. After three months of medical treatment, we could start to wean him off the medication, while continuing with environmental adjustments. After six months, Lucifer was no longer on any medication at all. Huguette's apartment was well outfitted to meet the needs of the cat, who had recovered his balance, his ability to adapt. Lucifer had learned how to control his claws so much better: he still exercised his talents as a predator, but only on objects that were meant for him. Huguette and her plant spray bottle removed all risk of attack thanks to her perfect timing. Within a few weeks, she no longer needed to live with her spray bottle constantly at hand.

They were finally living in harmony, and the treatment came to an end: Huguette knew that if the "aggressions" started up again, there were solutions; and she had spread the word. She told me, most amused, that she had said to her doctor that she was glad not to have taken his advice to abandon her cat, as there were other solutions that were more respectful of the animal and the bond between them. Not all such stories have a happy ending (as you will remember with Nougat), but good results of this kind encourage us vets to continue our work focused on the well-being of both cats and humans.

Nougatine and Catherine: Treating Mood Problems

Certain feline patients accompanied by an extraordinary human can teach us a lot as vets: their role is to instruct us in the fundamental elements of our practice; ours is to discover new ways of caring for them. If Prima was a big influence on me in teaching me how to handle cats, Nougatine and Catherine were significant milestones in my treatment of behavioral illnesses in cats.

Nougatine was the first case of cat bipolar dysthymia that I diagnosed, treated, and followed up on over the course of many years. This cat opened the door for me on what cat madness could look like, while her owner showed me how empathy, patience, and fierce determination made it possible to live with a cat with a serious condition of this kind.

At that time, I was a general practitioner in Toulon and, once or twice a month, I would spend my Thursdays off holding consultations in veterinary psychiatry in and around Nice. I mainly practiced in clinics but, in certain cases, I visited the client's home. One evening in August, in the lovely Musicians Quarter, I made the acquaintance of Nougatine, a young female Siamese with puzzling behavioral issues. This case dates from a while ago, and Nougatine is no longer with us, but it has remained engraved in my memory. When I visited them at home, the family, with my client Catherine taking the lead, described to me moments of tension and the surprise attacks Nougatine would make in very precise circumstances.

When I saw her, the cat was going through one of her "bad spells"; there had been a number of aggressive incidents in the previous few days. I sat at the kitchen table, and, after a few minutes, Nougatine leaped onto my lap. "Be careful, the slightest movement on your part might set off an attack," Catherine had warned me. Sometimes, clients enjoy winding you up by exaggerating how aggressive their animal is, but that wasn't the case here. The young cat who had jumped onto my knee was quivering, taut as a piano string, and I knew the threat was real. In a similar case I'd dealt with, when the crisis came and the slightest movement could set the cat off, it would perch on the dresser above the kitchen table. "No one move. Put your cutlery on the table and don't move a muscle," the father of the family would warn. The cat had attacked, painfully, on a number of occasions, and the family had learned that only total stillness lessened the risk.

Nougatine wasn't quite as dangerous as that, but her attacks could be pretty lethal nonetheless. Anyone who hasn't lived with an animal suffering from this type of condition may find it hard to understand. The classic advice from those around you is to get rid of the cat and the danger at the same time. In some cases, that will be the only solution, but as Nougatine and a few others have shown, there is another way. Treating bipolar dysthymia in a cat (see box) requires patience and prudence.

Major Behavioral Instability: A Symptom of Bipolar Problems

Bipolar dysthymia in cats is a fairly close equivalent of the human bipolar condition: a mood disorder that can be triggered by certain elements in the environment or sometimes without there being any specific cause of the crisis. Living with an animal that suffers from this condition can be worrying as it may behave in unpredictable ways. Charming one minute, displaying normal behavior (such as demanding to be stroked and other displays of affection), it can change in an instant into a wildcat, attacking anyone close by, its eyes bulging and with no control over its claws or its bite.

In the absence of any treatment for a cat so affected, the whole family has to be quite determined to keep such a pet. Happily, these days, after much trial and error, some medications have been found that seem to have a moderate but persistent effect on these problems. We can't say that an animal suffering from bipolar dysthymia will be able to be cured absolutely and definitively. It will always be fragile. Nevertheless, when the family is on board, then one is able to treat these animals, which can lead to greater predictability. Though the illness is described as unpredictable, it is usually not difficult to identify what is known as an aura phase—that is, warning signs indicating that a crisis is in the offing and the cat is about to become dangerous. At that point, there is no question of controlling the cat, of attempting to take charge of it. The only option is to get it, and yourself, out of the way, usually by shutting it in a room without visual or auditory stimulation, in order to minimize anything that could exacerbate the crisis—a bit like dealing with someone who is having an epileptic fit. It's quite similar, in fact: the crisis may have an internal cause, but many external factors can aggravate it.

One of the greatest medical mistakes of the last century was to try to separate neurology and psychiatry: they both target the same organ, and sometimes the distinction between the two is somewhat tenuous. It was not so long ago that there was a discipline known as neuropsychiatry. It had no doubt become too large not to be subdivided, but it was primarily psychoanalysis that encouraged the viewing of body and mind as separate entities. It is fortunate that animals can't speak, which has prevented vets from taking this approach, and so we haven't lost track of the close connection of the brain with the rest of the body.

Nougatine and Catherine Forever

When I saw Nougatine, the discipline was in its infancy, and we were taking the first faltering steps in treating complicated cases like this. Catherine, her owner, was infinitely patient not only with her cat but also with this young vet who was doing his best to find a course of treatment that would make her life livable. I still find it remarkable that, once a diagnosis is established and we can give the condition a name, the owners become significantly less anxious. It isn't some weird unknown thing but an identifiable illness that their cat is suffering from. Quite recently I learned an extraordinary lesson from an owner who contacted me during the first Covid lockdown for a telephone consultation as she couldn't find anyone locally to take care of her dog, which was presenting symptoms of bipolarity. It turned out that this lady was a psychiatric nurse, and when I chatted with her on the phone, she said: "You know, I think I know what my animal is suffering from, and everyone I have talked to about it has said, 'There is only one solution—you need to have him put down.' Would you believe it? Suppose we treated humans the same way, suppose we performed euthanasia on every bipolar person. I find it hard to believe that animals can't benefit from the same medical treatments as humans."

I share that opinion. I know that this will shock those who think that there is an impenetrable barrier between animals and people and that it is unthinkable that we should offer them the same level of care. For philosophical or religious reasons, some people find this solidarity of care for mental illness intolerable to contemplate. I leave them to their certainties: it's the opposite that I find shocking. Sometimes the limit is technical: we don't have the medication or the knowledge or we don't have the procedures for controlling a disorder, and, in very severe cases, where the family itself is endangered, with a heavy heart, we may be forced to give up. But often we can attempt a treatment with the consent of all concerned. This was the case with Nougatine.

At that time I was testing a product that claimed to be a mood stabilizer. The trials we were running were aimed at dogs and some of their anxiety issues. I have to stress that there were very few products in the vet's pharmacopoeia in those days designed especially for cats, and I don't mean psychotropics, which didn't exist at all in a cat-specific form. It was published research on the part of experts and in particular the consent of cat owners that gave us permission—in the equivalent of a compassionate-use protocol—to diverge from the beaten track. Dysthymic disorders, as the name suggests, are mood problems such as depression (certain forms of which are known as dysthymia in human medicine).

With Catherine's agreement, I treated Nougatine with selegiline, a mood stabilizer, anxiolytic, and neuron protector, emphasizing that there was no guarantee of success. I wasn't the first to try to help Nougatine. The vets who had treated her in general practice were among the very few practitioners at the time who were interested in behavioral disorders, and they had tried some drug-based approaches. Benzodiazepines and morphine had no effect or, on the contrary, merely aggravated the behavioral problems when crises occurred. Nougatine displayed some spectacular symptoms: rolling skin syndrome (RSS), or twitchy cat disease; violent tail wagging as a crisis approached; and asomatognosia (when a cat doesn't recognize its own tail and starts to attack it). These are all ways in which a cat may express suffering during episodes that are painful physically and psychologically.

Once the diagnosis has been established, the underlying mechanisms of the crises are explicable: there is no need for owners to feel guilty as they realize that their cat's illness has nothing to do with them and they can help their pet without feeling responsible for its problems. In this case, the family had lost a cat not long before they acquired Nougatine. "We are too invested," Catherine told me. There can be issues with dogs and cats that are acquired as replacements, but I have never known bipolar dysthymia to be caused by that. No blame need be attached as there is no other cause than the illness itself.

I offered a compassionate treatment: the mysterious selegiline comes in tablet form, very difficult for a cat to swallow, but Catherine and her family would manage somehow. I have learned over many years that, with the right motivation, these obstacles can be surmounted and ingenious solutions can be found, even if cats are not always cooperative in receiving medical treatment.

Nougatine took her medicine and she got better. That doesn't mean she was cured. A visit from a grandniece triggered new crises, even when everything seemed to be going well. "It used to be impossible; now it's tolerable," Catherine observed philosophically at a follow-up appointment. We all like to hear about glorious triumphs, but given the deep-seated nature of psychological issues, this was all highly optimistic. That is to say, we won the right to continue caring for Nougatine, to find the course of treatment most likely to provide the best quality of life for the cat and its group.

I continued to receive news of Nougatine for a long time: she lived a full cat life with her illness more or less under control, surrounded by understanding and love that she returned unconditionally. There are more and more of us who share Catherine's conviction: we can't cure everything, but that doesn't stop us providing treatment, to be there as a companion, and to make life possible in many cases that might have felt desperate.

Later on we will encounter other cases, other cats, and discover that there is a specific feline psychiatric pathology, as has already been established in dogs.

2

Territorial Problems

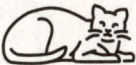

I love cats because I love my house and they gradually become its visible soul.

—Jean Cocteau

Here we are, then, with a barely tamed predator who can sometimes revert to being wild. Yet we like living together and—in the vast majority of cases—don't want to give up on this precious cohabitation. Sharing your house with cats means embracing otherness. We learn that it is possible to live in harmony with very different beings as long as we respect the "other" in all its strangeness and are able to agree on areas of mutual benefit, in which the surprising, shared pleasure of the encounter plays no small part.

This involves sharing a living space. So this will be the second stage of our journey, the second key to entering the world of cats: their well-being depends on the harmony of their habitat, their ability to organize it according to their needs while adhering to certain fundamental principles. Their habitat is also at the root of many problems.

Princess Choupette

According to her owner, Carole, Choupette was a princess.

They lived in an apartment in the suburbs of Paris where Carole's daughter sometimes came to stay. All was going well: they shared moments of tenderness; their life together was well organized. Choupette often slept on her owner's bed, or on a shelf in a cupboard. She was very clean: she did her business in a litter box.

And then came the first Covid lockdown. To make it more bearable, Carole decided to go and stay in her parents' house in the south of France. They would have a lot more space. Her daughter came too, as well as her son with his girlfriend and another friend. After a few days, and much to the chagrin of Carole, who was worried about her mother's house being damaged, Choupette started making messes around the place. She urinated on a bed, then on the couch, then on an armchair. Not a princess anymore.

Carol had a theory that could prove to be useful: the cat had been stressed by the hasty move to the new house. Encountering new human cohabitants might also have upset her. The son was neither a familiar nor soothing figure for the cat, according to his mother. However, the cat's medical history did not indicate an anxious state, and what Choupette was doing was unwanted urination, not marking.

Let's Be Precise

Let's pause a moment to explain this. It is fundamental to the diagnosis. When a client arrives complaining that their cat is unclean, this in fact tells us nothing unless we ask further questions. By asking five questions (see table), it is nearly always possible to distinguish changed, unwanted urination from marking.

Distinguishing Unwanted Urination from Marking		
	Unwanted urination	Marking
Posture	Crouched	Standing
Surface	Horizontal	Vertical
Volume	Heavy	Light
Vocalization	Absent	Present
Sequence	Regular urination (*sniffs the ground, scratches, turns around, crouches, urinates in silence, scratches, covers, checks*)	Marking (*exhibits flehmen response, turns around, tail erect, discharges a jet of urine while emitting a particular sound, then leaves*)

Urination is a moment of vulnerability for cats: they have to be silent and precise to cover up their traces. Marking is a signal directed at other cats: it combines several channels of communication.

This is not a theoretical distinction: unwanted urination goes hand in hand with an anxious state, and we have to identify the cause. It occurs above all when the usual zone of urination has changed and become inaccessible to the cat.

In Choupette's case, we were in the first lockdown, so I had to arrange an online consultation. As we were speaking, the cat climbed onto the armchair in front of Carole and performed a perfect urination sequence. This technology, which we are now allowed to use under certain conditions, enables us to witness behaviors when previously at best we had to rely on what the cat's owner told us. I asked Carole to give me a video tour of the house, principally the spots where the cat slept, ate her food, observed, and interacted, in addition to the urination area.

Seeing the bathroom where the litter box was located provided us with the solution. In the rushed departure from Paris, no one thought to bring the bag of the cat's usual and preferred litter. Carole had quickly found a substitute, but it hadn't suited Choupette. A case of the princess and the pea? Not exactly.

The organization of its living space is a central element in a cat's equilibrium, a nonnegotiable aspect of its needs. It doesn't stamp its feet, demanding a product that it likes better; rather, the major zones of its environment have become disorganized, which throws it off balance.

When we managed to find the right litter for Choupette, we added a food supplement to her anti-anxiety anxiolytic medication to make sure that the changes to her surroundings didn't trigger an emotional imbalance and to limit the risk that a recurrent state of anxiety would become a fixed pattern of behavior. Carole didn't even need to administer it: as soon as the litter box reacquired its familiar characteristics for the cat, the cleanliness problem disappeared.

A Mirror of Our Values

These days, some people see their cats as royalty, whereas the cats themselves probably have no such aspirations.[1] The more we vets see of cats, the more the things people say about them seem disrespectful of their species: we should not project our human faults and qualities onto them (anthropomorphism) nor judge them only by the yardstick of what humans are capable of, thereby relegating all other species to an inferior status (anthropocentrism). I try to avoid these two pitfalls, while also trying to make the world of cats accessible by comparing it to our own. We should bear in mind Wittgenstein's words about another big cat: "If a lion could talk, we wouldn't be able to understand him." We humans spend our time interpreting what we see according to our belief systems, points of reference, and values. Cats have paid a price for this: at times their strange behavior has been seen as the work of the devil or witches. Nowadays, when this very same behavior chimes in with the values of our age, cats are instead revered as icons.

Cats may not be kings but they are well on the way to winning the popularity contest among domestic animals (in fact, in France and Germany they already have). When I started out in professional practice in the late 1980s, France had more than 10 million dogs and fewer than 8 million cats. Today, in the early 2020s, with 15 million cats, France is the country with the largest ratio of cats to humans, at 1:5; in particular, the number of domestic felines is more than double that of dogs (15.2 million cats compared to 7.2 million dogs). This is not the case anywhere else. The craze for cats is shared across the world, but it is striking that in France this is to the detriment of dogs. In the UK approximately 12 million dogs are kept as pets, compared to 11 million cats. In the US there are nearly 77 million dogs and 59 million cats.

Two factors have contributed to this peaceful feline invasion: The cat is tailor-made for the internet. And it perfectly fits in with our new way of living.

Internet Star

The first reason for this is an aesthetic one. It has to be said: you can't get much cuter than a kitten, and they have become stars of the internet. This sometimes drives vets to despair, when posts of helpful therapeutic information and news of scientific developments sink without a trace while a picture of a litter of kittens drives a lot of traffic to their websites. Even adult cats get some of the glory. Chances are you have heard of Tardar Sauce, a.k.a. "Grumpy Cat." The brother of the owner, Tabatha Bundesen, was a photographer who posted images of the cat online, which became a meme with captions based on the cat's curmudgeonly demeanor.

Grumpy Cat was all about expressing contempt, even hatred, for humans to the amusement of millions of internet users all around the world. But this wasn't just a question of a viral meme; there was big money involved. The cat's owner has never confirmed it, but it is believed that Grumpy Cat has earned around $100 million from advertising, merchandising, and a plagiarism lawsuit.[2] It is unfortunate that the messages she was asked to convey were such misanthropic ones. One of the last that I saw, long after the cat's death, said: "It's official: cats don't transmit Covid, but they would if they could." I can be as amused as the next person while regretting their effect on how cats are perceived.

Why This Craze?

The respective rise and fall in cat and dog ownership in France can be explained by changes in lifestyle. The Covid-19 pandemic changed many things, and the sense I get from my colleagues is that it is due to a craze for both species rather than an overwhelming majority of cat adoptions or purchases since the lockdowns. If we rewind to the start of the 2020s, what do we find? Many people live in small homes, increasingly in the center of cities, and can't imagine ever owning a dog. But this overlooks the desire, the need, felt by many people for the companionship of an animal as a pet: it holds out the promise, almost always fulfilled, of affection, tenderness, and even love. Having a pet by your side can improve your health and your life in general and give you a greater sense of purpose. That may seem a little clichéd, but we can cite hundreds of scientific publications in support of this; a recent overview of the literature backs the notion that owning a dog, for instance, can increase feelings of hopefulness.[3]

There isn't so much literature on the benefits of cats. Of course, cats don't need to be walked and so do not create opportunities for more social contact: when scientists tried to measure the impact on well-being and mood, it was therefore the effect of the relationship that they assessed. We don't have the same relationships with cats as we do with dogs. That might appear obvious, but it has been the source of many misunderstandings. For example, numerous studies have been skewed by including elements that are only relevant to a relationship with dogs.[4] People who have adopted or bought cats by default, because they think they wouldn't be able to own a dog but are expecting the same thing, risk being disappointed.

In any case, urbanization has influenced the increase in the number of domestic felines. But why is France the only country where there is such a marked difference between the number of cats and dogs? As well as choosing their pets to fit the places in which they live, the French also do so in relation to their working conditions. We have more days of vacation than any other country in Europe, and even before the pandemic, the reduction in working time, whether measured in hours or days, encouraged taking time off and short vacation breaks that can be difficult to organize (or very expensive) with a dog, while with a cat an automatic food dispenser and a clean litter box allow you to go off for two or three days at a time without, in most cases, any adverse consequences for your kitty.

As well as being beautiful, cats are thus also a practical choice of pet. However, more and more cats present behavioral symptoms when they are left for too long on their own: compulsive licking that removes all the fur from their tail or belly; fecal or urinary soiling; changes in urinary marking—all increasingly common signs that indicate how regularity in the relationship is a major factor for cats.

Last but not least, and this is probably the most important thing, cats are in step with key modern values, such as body consciousness (another key that we will explore later) and "cocooning"—the attention we pay to the interior of our homes to create havens of peace and a psychic resource. This impulse brings us closer to cats, who have been practicing this art for millennia.

Homeland Security

While cats may not be our rulers, to our eyes they seem to be staking out their living space as if they own it and then lording over it, which suggests solemnity and power. But let's avoid such errors of interpretation and stick to using our keys to understanding cats. You will remember the first key I gave you: cats are both predator and prey at the same time.

Now you have a second key: the place where they live is of paramount importance. Let us try to think like a cat and follow the thread that guides us through the labyrinth of their minds. I will often invite you to try to put yourself in a cat's place, not to think like a human pretending to be a cat, but to see the world through the eyes, brain, emotions, and cognitions of a cat. It's difficult, virtually impossible. To think like a cat we would have to see, hear, feel like one. We would have to have whiskers and be able to process the information they provide. But, as you will see, with a bit of training you will be able to put yourself in the place of your pet cat. Your cat may not be a king on his throne, but the insights you will gain will be all the more fascinating for that.

Prey and predator, equipped with different senses and adapted to its duality, the cat always organizes its living place to cope with all the exigencies of this double nature: so that it can both protect itself and hunt.

In the clinical cases I describe, it is very often a disruption of the harmony between these two poles that creates an imbalance. This triggers clinical symptoms: the cat expressing its inability to reorganize its territory in a satisfactory manner.

Let us from the outset nail a point of dispute between scientists. I will repeatedly use the word "territory," but it should be understood in an everyday sense and not in its ethological meaning. A territorial species is defined as one that defends all parts of its territory, especially against members of its own species, except for its sexual partner and its offspring. This is not the case with the space occupied by a domestic cat: many cats are indeed able to defend—quite successfully—certain parts of their environment, but this does not apply to the whole of the space they occupy. On the contrary, they might like sharing certain parts of that environment at certain moments for games, for cuddles—in short, for a whole range of interactions that mean that they cannot be regarded as a territorial species.

It is high time that we changed our understanding of this notion of territoriality and applied a little nuance. The work of the Belgian philosopher Vinciane Despret on birds has a lot of resonance with our current work of redefining the notion of territory.[5] To paraphrase her, I would say: "When we talk about cats we must stop thinking like suburban homeowners." Vets in my field sometimes talk about territory in the sense of living space, biotope, home range. For us, such expressions all refer to the same thing, and even if the word "territory" slips out in these pages, it is not meant to be restricted to a narrow definition of a territorial space.

The foundation of a balanced life for a cat is a living place that allows it to feel secure as well as to explore, observe, and hunt. But then, if all that is necessary, is it possible to keep a cat in an apartment without contravening such fundamental rules and without seeing it as captive, a mistreated animal denied the means to express its natural behavior?

We can now answer that with a categorical yes. A cat can be perfectly well-balanced living inside an apartment if it can find the necessary resources there. Rest assured, it isn't very complicated to create the right conditions, and the vast majority of cats I see in my practice lead happy lives, filled with everything they need.

Now, this feeling, shared by many practitioners, is evidently not proof. We will discuss this in more detail later on, but for now let us note that a number of publications and much of the research carried out as part of my university degree in veterinary psychiatry have established that there is no difference in prevalence of behavioral problems between cats who are able to go outside and those who can't.

Five Fundamental Needs

For now, I invite you to understand how a cat's biotope (or habitat) is put together. Remember the number five. It is almost a magic number for understanding cats.

They organize their world into different zones. Whatever their normal environment, inside or outside, in a cage at the clinic or at large in wide-open fields, it is possible to identify five zones that correspond to five fundamental needs (see box).

The Five Zones of a Cat's World

Isolation: Where the cat sleeps, grooms itself, and where it will feel most safe.

Feeding: Where it will find its food.

Disposal: A carefully chosen place where it can defecate and urinate in complete safety, and the source of much quid pro quo with humans.

(Solitary) activities: Where the cat can spend a lot of time observing, hunting, and playing with no need of partners.

Interactions: Where interactions—although they aren't essential—can be sought and appreciated by our domestic feline. These usually happen in particular places and at precise moments.

These zones are interconnected by invariable routes marked out with distinctive pheromones. This is very specific to cats: alongside their main olfactory system they have a supplementary one purely for the detection of pheromones (see box on p. 77). A feline's territory is organized according to its five senses with an extra command center: olfaction in its two forms. There is also a time element to this. Certain spots around the house can never serve as a zone of isolation in the morning but may be happily used as such in the afternoon. Such zones tell us a lot about a cat's behavioral balance based on where they are, how permanent they are, and how they're distributed.

Let us take a closer look at the detail. If you have a cat, find some paper and try to draw the map of your cat's biotope: you will see that it will explain many of your pet's behaviors.

Zone of Isolation: Panic Room

Think like a cat: in order to rest and to do your grooming—two moments when you can't be on your guard as much as you might have to—you need somewhere very secure when you are in prey mode. If you are in predator mode, by contrast, or simply in the mode of "I don't sense any danger nearby," then you can stretch out in the open, in a place that is accessible to others whom you don't consider a danger.

What is your cat's favorite spot for the night or for its long siestas? Figaro always perched on top of a cupboard in a rather large perforated pot that offered him a perfect hiding place while still allowing him to keep an eye on his surroundings, whereas Tounet chose a rocking chair in a room that was quiet but accessible. As for the cats who have shared my life, mysterious Hermione always hid away to rest, Chiquita plonked herself on the middle of the sofa, and Galy, the little Sphynx, could sleep on my computer between me and the screen. Nowadays, Flora, when she can, sleeps on me. She approaches with featherlight tread when I am asleep in bed and lies down on my back, while I pretend not to notice.

We have already touched on cats who suffer from HSHA, hyperactive animals. One of the keys to diagnosing this is disruption to the sleeping pattern. These cats sleep anywhere, even in the spot where they were playing just five minutes before. Parents of hyperactive children describe a similar phenomenon, the difficulty of putting their children to bed right up to the moment when, like the flicking of an off switch, they fall asleep wherever they happen to be.[6]

For a few months I looked after Rammus, my son's ginger cat. The diagnosis of HSHA was unambiguous, and the treatment saved the cat's life. I mention him here because he was a chaotic and amusing illustration of the hyperactive cat's inability to make a zone of isolation like other cats.

I have photos of Rammus fast asleep in the middle of my son's living room, on the floor. You don't do that if you want to be a little out of the way. Anyone might turn up, jump on you, or injure you. As his treatment progressed, Rammus learned that a zone of isolation needed to tick certain boxes: he chose places that were high up but still well exposed, such as the dining-room table, weight-training bench, or ironing board; then he raised his sights again and slept in places that no cat before him in the house had used. On top of the kitchen cupboards, more than six feet up, became one of his favorite places. Every now and again I would feel I was being observed and would look up to see him staring at me, a pair of watchful eyes beneath the two small pointed triangles of his ears.

Eventually, as Rammus made progress, he rediscovered the need to feel enclosed and protected. He tried the laundry basket, which sat atop the ironing board. It's a classic spot for many cats and a nightmare for anyone who comes to sort the clean laundry and finds it covered in cat hair. Chased out of the laundry basket, he found his way to different sinks. I found him curled up in a ball in the bathroom sink on more than one occasion, and when I made it clear to him that I wanted to use it and so his nest was about to be filled with water, he'd give me such a reproachful look at times that I would leave him in peace and go off to find another place to brush my teeth. Then there were the cupboards, but inside this time. It was easy to tell when he had found a new location from the pile of clothes he'd displaced onto the floor. After that experience with Rammus I always asked owners about their cat's zone of isolation and followed up on it when treating HSHA. While hyperactive cats will fail to select a regular and peaceful zone of isolation, anxious cats, by contrast, will always look for the most protected and hidden-away place possible, which they won't want to share. At least, in most cases. But generalizing can lead us astray, and it could be something else. Some owners say, for instance, how their cat can only sleep on them, on their chest or head. As vets, we then look for signs of autonomopathy, whereby an adult animal is prevented from achieving full independence, leaving it reliant on the attachment figure always being present. Sometimes it's just a choice on the part of the cat, but that needs to be checked. All in all, the places chosen by our cats tell us a lot about their emotional balance.

Zone of Feeding: Delicatessen

Our domestic cats are commensals: they benefit from our food without harming us. This is the case when we don't let them hunt for food. Otherwise, they could very well be self-sufficient. When we control their food, three points have to be taken into consideration: the place where they eat, which should be protected and allow them to feed undisturbed; the frequency with which they eat; and the type of food they enjoy.

Once again, we have to forget what we know about ourselves, we have to forget what we know about dogs, and try to enter the mind of this small feline, at once prey and predator. In a natural environment, a cat spends a lot of its time hunting. Then it is on the lookout and very vigilant. It is in hunter mode and protection mode at the same time. It can stay for hours watching a hole into which it has seen a small field mouse or vole disappear, waiting to grab it when it reappears. A cat can also watch birds for long periods at a time, hoping to catch one, with only a very slim likelihood of success. According to the classic ethological works, a cat consumes the equivalent of a small mouse between ten and fifteen times a day.[7]

Why this regular snacking on small prey rather than doing what their big cousin the lion does and hunting a large animal that will keep it satiated for days on end? You may have guessed the answer. What do lions do after their copious meals? They digest while sleeping, with no risk of being attacked in their sleep. This isn't the case with a cat: it is much safer to have small meals and several short naps in well-protected places than to be exposed and unconscious for too long, where it could be discovered by another predator. Its double nature as prey–predator is once again key to understanding this behavior.

This raises another question: Can we respond to this animal's needs if we live in an apartment? Of course we can. By dividing up the distribution of food, we can satisfy this primal need. It is a common cause of behavioral dysfunction that is luckily easy to put right once it is discovered. Let us consider Coquin, a beautiful black house cat who was brought to me for a consultation after losing a large amount of fur from his belly and the back of his legs—what we call *extensive feline alopecia*. Coquin was a nice cat and fairly potbellied, which didn't suggest that there was any lack of feeding involved—and yet . . .

He had been seen by his usual vet, who referred him to a specialist in dermatology. The most common cause of feline alopecia is fleas, and an allergic reaction to their saliva. He was given a thorough checkup: there were no fleas; nor was there any bacterial or fungal infection. This is usually the point at which behavioral issues are then considered. When we examine such cats with a dermatoscope, we see a healthy skin and alopecia in the form of a self-inflicted absence of fur. It is the cat's exaggerated, compulsive licking that has removed the fur. The hairs are cropped very short, as if sliced at the root by very sharp scissors. The cat's taste buds on its tongue act as a grater and cut the hair at the base, in a compulsive licking unchecked by any stop mechanism. This licking is in fact a displacement activity and an important marker of anxiety. Hyperphagia, an abnormally increased appetite for food, is another such marker. With Coquin, the two activities had consequences: moderate obesity and much more serious alopecia. He was suffering from a state of anxiety, but we didn't yet understand the cause. Etiological investigation is always a delicate but exciting part of a consultation: this is when we try to get inside the heads of our feline patients and of the humans who accompany them.

Alain and Jacqueline loved Coquin and they wanted to look after him properly. Searching for the one detail that would make everything click into place, I suddenly grasped a fundamental point.

"How do you feed Coquin?"

"We've always had animals and we do it the same way as we've done with them."

"Were your other animals also cats?"

"Ah, no. We've only had dogs before."

"And how often do you feed him?"

"Once a day, like we've always done."

The aim wasn't to point out mistakes but to get to the cause of the anxious state. Cats are not small dogs—this bears repeating, and Coquin was further proof of that.

I saw Coquin in May, and he didn't have a hair on his belly; I saw him again in August, and all his bare areas were covered again in lovely black fur. I supplemented the rebalancing of food distribution with a nutraceutical that was very efficient in controlling anxiety in cats. In cases such as this, once the cause is discovered, the cure is well established.

Don't forget that, for the sake of its well-being, a cat must eat several times a day. Sometimes, discovering the cause of the problem is a more subtle matter: the food regime is responsible, but it is not the distribution that is the root of the problem but the type of food. Some cats prefer dried food such as kibble. Others prefer wet food. If you live with a cat, you get to know what its needs are and also its tastes.

I was contacted by a colleague concerning the cat at her veterinary clinic, a mascot cat of the sort that are very common. Vets are very often moved by a cute face or a touching story. Biscotte had ended up in this clinic after being brought in by firefighters. He came in with a very damaged eye and in poor physical shape. After pepping him up and removing the injured eye, the clinic workers bonded with him, and Biscotte became a fixture, with license to roam all over the clinic. He became a bit of a star, making friends with humans and animals alike. If a dog barked at him as he walked by, he gave it a wide berth, but he never spat or scratched: a real sweetie. He had just one fault: he raided the bags of kibble that were for sale. After a few weeks he was denied access to the storeroom and the display room. Needless to say, there was some excellent-quality kibble at his disposal. After a few more weeks, a bit like Coquin, Biscotte began licking his belly so hard that he pulled out all the fur.

An excellent general practitioner with a keen interest in dermatology and animal behavior, my colleague pursued several lines of inquiry. Fleas? No. An allergy would have been reduced by cortisone treatment, but that didn't work. She then considered a lack of self-control, as in HSHA, which can turn animals into thieves with an insatiable appetite. That would be somewhat surprising, as the other signs were not present: no hypersensitivity, no mad running about. The cat wasn't leaping about, reacting to everything. He slept well, in suitable zones of isolation, and he controlled his claws and teeth except on the aforementioned bags of kibble, which were all ripped open but the contents never consumed.

Unsurprisingly, the treatment for hyperactivity resulted in no improvement. The hypothesis of an anxious state, connected to the barred access and hence modification of the cat's biotope, was another reasonable line of inquiry. Treatment and enrichment of the environment did not result in any improvement. Biscotte was always gentle and friendly, but he had no belly fur left and was still opening any bags he could get his teeth into.

It is always difficult to intervene after so many unsuccessful attempts. Summoned in to help, I tried to understand what might be going on in the cat's head. He had been brought in by the firefighters and his exact age was unknown, but it was possible that he had spent several weeks in contact with his mother. Female cats inculcate many things in their kittens: how to cover their traces, how to hide up high, and also how to hunt. When they are able to, the mother cat brings dead prey when the kittens are around six or seven weeks, and then, three weeks later, she brings live prey. This is designed to teach familiarity with prey and hunting techniques. For some kittens who have received this teaching, nothing ever replaces prey.

What set me thinking was the fact that this cat was interested in blood tests. This is not exactly a common proclivity— after all, you have to be a vet's cat to be able to indulge it. Suddenly the symptom of opening a bag of kibble without consuming the contents potentially made sense. We told ourselves that we needed to go further in the work of achieving empathy with the cat. What motivated him to open several bags without consuming what he managed to obtain? Once the bag was open, he could have eaten a lot of kibble, which is what a hyperactive cat would have done. But Biscotte simply went and opened another. This is what gave us the idea that what this cat lacked was in fact access to wet food, food that better reminded him of prey than kibble did. I agreed with my colleague that seven or eight times a day we would give him some wet food that best matched his tastes and at the same time a strong dose of an anti-anxiety product derived from milk. After a few weeks of this double treatment, wet food distributed often with a nutraceutical, I received a phone call telling me that Biscotte had stopped licking himself and that his fur was starting to grow back.

Eating in every facet of the activity is fundamental for a cat, and it is not just about the place (the zone of feeding), but also and above all the frequency of meals and sometimes, as was the case here, the very nature of the food itself.

Zone of Disposal: The Need for Cleanliness

Cats have a reputation for cleanliness—a reputation that is well deserved. Anyone who has acquired a puppy or a kitten at the age of eight weeks, the minimum age, will know the difference. With a puppy, you have two or three months' work still ahead of you to get it house-trained, but there is every chance that your kitten will arrive already clean. Why do cats have this ability? Why the rapid learning process? In dogs, a social species, at most the learning will consist of not doing their business in their sleeping place and using designated spaces.

With the kitten, the mother plays a proactive part in its learning. She shows her kittens how to find a good spot, scratch, and bury, breaking the sequence down into stages and checking that she has the attention of all her young students. This learning through imitation is not just random; the mothers give "lessons" at the moments when the kittens are interested in them: lessons in disposing of waste, in self-control, in grooming, in climbing—everything that prey needs to escape its potential aggressors.

When it comes to using a litter box, remember that we are talking about disposal and not marking. We have already discussed the difference between these two behaviors. The same key will serve to open the door to understanding. A cat is vulnerable when it is doing its business, and the smell of its excrement can alert predators. It is therefore crucial for the cat to cover its excrement and check that it is leaving as little olfactory trace as possible. That is why, if you observe your cat, you will see it first of all choose its spot, sniff at it sometimes for quite a long time, turn around, crouch, defecate into the hollow it has thus created, then turn around again. Covering up and smelling again: often it's not enough and the cat will add another layer of litter before walking away. This is the normal sequence of disposal. It can vary somewhat according to the personality of each cat. Some are very meticulous, others much more negligent, and a behavioral issue can upset the sequence of disposal in a major way. It is easy to imagine our hyperactive friend not being very attentive to the way in which it covers up its excrement. It will jump into its box, quickly do its business, scratch around in a way that is as intense as it is ineffective—that is, without covering its traces but managing to scatter cat litter all around the box. Then it will run away. The phobic cat, by contrast, will not tolerate its box being soiled in the slightest way.

So many cats, so many forms of disposal, but a few rules might help us to offer our felines the best possible zone of disposal. It may seem trivial to pay this much attention to litter. But when you understand the importance for a cat of its zone of disposal, then it becomes crucial to work out all the elements that can upset it and set off inappropriate and undesirable forms of disposal outside the box. In these cases, the cat will choose a spot that suits it: a piece of furniture where it can scratch and cover, a plant pot, or the bed with its duvet might serve as favored alternatives, albeit ones that the owners won't be very pleased about.

The Litter Box

To work, it should meet four easy-to-remember requirements that relate to four major characteristics:

Capacity: It's a fact that cats have gotten bigger over the last few decades. The craze for larger breeds—such as the

Norwegian Forest cat or the Maine Coon—means that cats weigh an average of eleven pounds today compared with about eight pounds twenty years ago. The standard litter boxes you can buy in stores have not moved with the times, however, and that is a mistake. A good-quality box should be about one and a half times the length of the cat measured from its nose to the base of its tail. The cat should be able to turn around inside it and scratch. Many fecal accidents are due to the wrong size of box.

Content: The litter itself is of prime importance for the cat, and this depends on what it was used to when it was developing. We can say, thanks to a study by a student in veterinary psychiatry, that the majority of cats prefer mineral-based litter.[8] In addition, they will prefer certain types of litter over others, and each owner should get to know what their cat's preference is. If in doubt, the best bet is to get a type of litter with the finest granules possible. Cats love earth, which explains why plant pots may provide an acceptable second choice. Often, the addition of a few plant beads will stop them from being used.

Location: Away from the cat's food and from their sleeping place. The box should be situated in a calm space that is always accessible, where the cat can feel safe taking the risk of being vulnerable without being threatened or disturbed. Vets often encounter cleanliness issues in cats that may simply derive from the litter box being badly placed. Putting it in the bathroom can be a solution as long as the door is left open or the cat has access (via a cat flap, for example). Even if your cat gets along well with your dog, it may not want to share these moments. Brutus, a young and friendly Boxer, would always accompany Melody when she used her box, blowing into her fur while she crouched down. They played together the rest of the time and enjoyed a harmonious relationship, but at such a moment she didn't want to play, just to be left to evacuate in peace. The bedroom was out of bounds to the dog, so she chose the humans' bed to do her business in peace, carefully urinating or defecating into the folds of the sheets. All that was needed to sort out the situation was to close off the room where her litter box was located, even though the owners were worried that this might mean that both animals could no longer be kept together.

A Fixed Location: This might seem obvious, but sometimes I am surprised at how it doesn't always occur to people. I treated a group of four cats for cleanliness issues (and aggression between them). These cats were all named after philosophers; I forget the names of two of them, but it was the relationship between the other two, Plato and Socrates, that was the root of the problem (unlike their historical counterparts). Plato was a young cat, and very intrusive, whereas Socrates, who was older, did not like to be disturbed. Plato was a prankster who would rush at the other cats, pulling up only inches in front of them. The two others, who were very placid, would watch him without reacting, reject his challenge or his invitation to play, and go on their way. Socrates would instead hiss at the young upstart, but the situation did not deteriorate. Out of the goodness of their hearts, the owners, who had noticed that Socrates liked to be warm, moved the cats' sleeping baskets to where they would catch the sun. Aware that the litter boxes should be near the sleeping place, they also moved the boxes to a different room. Now, we may be very different from cats, but just imagine going into a room that is, in quite unpredictable ways, alternately your living room or your toilet.

This little act of kindness was the straw that broke the camel's back. Plato's anxious state got worse, and his aggressive rushing became more frequent and more intense, and now provoked retaliation from Socrates. We had to reestablish both the harmony and the stability of the biotope by assigning the litter boxes to a fixed location (there were three of these for four cats, which is a little less than the rule strictly advocates as it should be number of cats plus one) and by treating Socrates's anxiety and Plato's impulsiveness. After a few weeks, I don't know if they were back on speaking terms (we will see that cats are not very good when it comes to reconciliation), but at least peace was restored at home.

Cleaning the Litter Box

This is always a delicate question since everyone has their own ideas about hygiene and takes it amiss if they are thought to be lax in their standards of cleanliness.

As I say again and again, each cat is unique. This is even more the case than for dogs. Nevertheless, one can give broad guidelines for cleaning litter boxes. You should remove the stools as soon as possible after they have been deposited and *at least* once a day.

One astute study showed that cats are sensitive not just to the odor of their litter boxes but also to the sight of excrement. The researchers placed little plastic stools in the litter; they didn't smell but they were a perfect replica of something another cat might have left. It was found that 50 percent of cats wouldn't use a box when they could see that it might contain the feces of another cat.[9]

The litter should be completely changed once a week. You no doubt know a cat whose litter is changed only once every three weeks yet who still remains clean. We are talking here about cases of undesirable disposal, outside the litter box, where we seek to put in place an efficient minimal standard protocol in order to restore clean behavior.

There are a number of questions connected to this. Should you use an open or closed box? An American team tried to answer this question and concluded that there was no difference provided there was a standard protocol in place.[10] All well and good, but that is not how it works in real life. When a box is enclosed, the owner can't see the excrement that has been deposited and so is unaware of the state of the litter. So they tend to remove the stools less often and fail to clean the box with the desired regularity. I can understand the need of many owners not to have the litter box exposed. My advice to them is simple: stick to a very precise and very systematic cleaning protocol. Remember to lift the lid and check if there is any excrement. If you do this consistently, you have a good chance of helping your cat to achieve a satisfactory level of cleanliness.

In behavioral pathology, unwanted disposal is one of the main issues that is brought to our attention. Even if it is not very glamorous, even if some might consider it unnecessary to spend so much time trying to understand and construct a zone of disposal that is suitable for a cat, it is an important prerequisite for harmonious cohabitation. By following the simple rules that we have just outlined, we can reduce the risk of setting off unwanted disposal in the house by more than 50 percent. This is a major reason why domestic cats are abandoned.

Zone of Activities: Hunting

I have separated solitary activities from interactive ones because this is an important distinction when thinking about the behavioral repertoire of the cat.

Once its primary needs are met, once it feels fully protected, the cat can invent its own life, and its resources are almost infinite. When it feels safe, it will spend long periods looking out of the window or even inside the house, taking refuge in a cat hammock or a shoe box. And of course, above all, it will hunt.

Dogs are much more opportunistic—they are scavengers and are happy with carrion if it saves them the bother of hunting—whereas cats always try to ply their skills as a predator. Even the cutest little house cat needs to do that. We have already seen that it might chase the hands and feet of the humans it lives with if there is nothing else in its environment that allows it to exercise this form of behavior. But once it has an opportunity, whether it is to chase after genuine prey or a lure dangled in front of it, the cat will spend a big part of its day lurking and hunting.

Whether it's treats in a cat feeder or food scattered throughout the house, or small prey that the cat will watch, what is important is for the cat to be able to devote a sufficient portion of time to this vital activity. Observation time and solitary games are in the majority of cases connected activities, preparatory to or following from the act of hunting.

Some programs have had a lot of success by monitoring cats that have access to the outdoors using GPS, which showed that cats that went out were able to cover an area of 7,500 square feet on average. A number of scientific studies have established a correlation between urban density and the surface area covered, but, on average, a female explores up to 27 yards from the house and a male up to 110 yards.

Their skill as hunters raises the question of cats' impact on biodiversity. These days, many people would like to prevent cats from going out to stop them from attacking other species; many others, by contrast, believe that not letting a cat go outside is tantamount to mistreatment. Both positions rely to a great degree on myth. Based on observations in Australia, the cat is the designated culprit for attacks on wild animals. But that is overlooking the fact that it is not a native carnivore in

Australia and has thus caused many species of small marsupials to be endangered, helpless in the face of this formidable hunter. In France, a survey by the National Museum of Natural History, with the collaboration of voluntary researchers and cat owners, showed that the prey cats brought home was quite diverse, and no single species was especially endangered by cats. Other studies from around the world show very similar results: that cats can have a big impact, but only in the close vicinity of where they live.[11]

Zone of Interactions: A Measured Need

At the top of Maslow's pyramid, or hierarchy of needs, as applied to cats comes interaction—the relations between cats and other living creatures. We will devote the next chapter to it, as it is so important in feline behavioral pathology. After the issue of uncleanliness, it is the second most common complaint of owners. Cats don't need relationships and if these are imposed or feel uncomfortable, they can be a significant source of undesirable behaviors and pathological states.

What we do know for sure is that these interactions should not take place just anywhere. As they may be beneficial but not strictly necessary, they must be well prepared, predictable, and always positive. When it comes to human relationships, we do this without thinking about it, but when we want relations with our cats to go well, it's better to make an appointment. When there is attachment and respect in these encounters they are a source of much pleasure, but relations with other individuals, including those of their own species, can also be a major source of stress in a cat's life. To reiterate, cats are not social creatures, but nor do they seek absolute solitude. And it is this point that is different from the notion of a territorial space: there are areas where cats accept sharing and even where they seek out the company of other individuals with whom they have activities in common. It's not everywhere and it's not all the time, and this can be a source of misunderstanding between cats and those who live with them, humans or dogs, for whom constant cohabitation is more of a necessity than a trial.

Interior Design for Cats

Now we have what it takes to design a plan of the ideal living space for our domestic cats, and anyone who owns a cat can draw this new map reflecting an understanding of feline needs. We should understand the importance of zones dedicated to the cat's security as prey (isolation, feeding, disposal) and how its sense of well-being contributes to developing other activities, whether solitary or not.

Cats do not need property, but rather protection and harmony. For them nesting was already fashionable.

Ritualized Routes between Zones

With this new map, you will view your cat through new eyes. You know that being able to organize its living space is vital to a cat, but we don't live in the same sensory world, so I will ask you to carefully observe how your cat moves from one room to another, from one zone to another.

You will notice that your cat always uses the same routes, even inside an apartment. They may vary somewhat, but only marginally. I usually cite the example of two cats I have lived with, and whom you have already met: Chiquita and her daughter Hermione. They lived in our house with unlimited access to the outside, and we would see them turn up at mealtimes at one of the kitchen windows. Chiquita always came in through the window above the sink while Hermione chose the one above the countertop. I had seen it happen on numerous occasions and would describe it at conferences I attended. The day after one of these conferences, I was drinking a cup of coffee at the kitchen table when I saw each cat take the route of the other. For a moment, I thought that they had done it deliberately, until I remembered that when you make generalizations about cats, or even just a generalization about a cat (he always does that!), you set yourself up to be contradicted. Still, that should not prevent us from trying to understand and identify the main traits that allow us to pin down the personality of each cat and its vulnerabilities.

One of my clients was a Tarantino fan and named his cats Mr. Black and Mr. White. Mr. White, the one that was more prey-oriented, organized his habitat in a very cautious way: he chose a zone of isolation that was quite high up; his zone of disposal had to be impeccable, his food familiar and given at regular intervals. He had many solitary activities and only a few, not very robust interactions. Mr. Black, on the other hand, was much more predator than prey in his own mind and he invaded any space he was allowed into; he had a number of different sleeping places; he could tolerate a slightly soiled litter box; he ate many different types of food—in particular, he loved fruit. He hunted anything that resembled prey, but also bits of string, aluminum pellets. He was a pleasant companion, sometimes a bit intrusive, and seemed to enjoy contact, which he would often come in search of. If I've presented these two cats as caricatures, you will have already understood that there was every shade, not just of gray but of all the colors, between them, offering an infinity of different personalities.

Nevertheless, the vast majority of cats always use the same routes for getting around. A friend who bred Birman cats had built quite a large enclosure in his garden. After a few months, some paths had been trodden down, showing cat routes, some shared, others particular to certain cats as they formed a network connecting the different zones of all the cats that allowed them to organize this finite space into a number of personal biotopes. That brings us to another characteristic of cats: they don't live in the same sensory world as we do.

Organizing by Smell: In the Kingdom of Pheromones

Cats have a highly developed sense of smell (see box), though the difference here is more one of degree than of kind. But they also share a characteristic that is strange to us: their lifelong ability to detect and use pheromones to tag their territory and organize their relationships.

The Cat's Two Olfactory Systems

Principal olfactory system: This is much like ours, except that it is much more efficient, with five times the surface area and ten times the number of receptors. Cats use this very heightened sense to decide whether the food presented is edible or not, good for it or not, which explains why when a cat has rhinitis or a cold its appetite is reduced and it loses its ability to eat. One tip here: carefully clean your cat's nose with some warm water before presenting it with its food. Smell is a major sense in the life of a cat.

Secondary olfactory system: This is dedicated to the detection of pheromones. Here we enter unknown territory. I have sometimes outlined the importance of these molecules in the early phases of attachment.[12] In fact, appeasing pheromones exist in all species and are part of maternal recognition; they allow the infant to form a bond and identify with its species on the basis of this privileged relationship.

Most of us know about the power of sex pheromones, which dictate preference, attraction, and a predisposition to action that our brain always allows us to control, in principle, as is the case with most mammals. In cats, pheromones have another dimension: cats produce and detect a lot of them. In effect they have a facial pheromone complex, a pheromone-producing factory located on their cheeks, stretching from the corners of the mouth to the base of the ears.

Five types (yes, five again!) have been identified within this complex, labeled F_1 to F_5. At present, the actions of F_1 and F_5 are still unknown, though we do know more about the other three.

A Positive Sign

F_3 is the one that interests us vets the most. It is the pheromone of familiarization with the environment and inanimate objects. It is the one cats lay down when you see them rubbing their faces—how often they do this varying from cat to cat—on a doorway, the leg of a chair, or a table. These marks say: *I am in a safe place*, and rediscovering them induces a positive emotional response. Overzealous housework is thus anathema to a cat, and cats and cleaners often find themselves in opposing camps. I recall one very beautiful house occupied by a family with a taste for fine minimalist Italian furnishings, including the kitchen with its resplendent tiles and lacquered surfaces looking as though they'd come straight out of a magazine. This kitchen was one of the few rooms accessible to the cat, which had been confined to the storeroom and the kitchen, having developed the bad habit, in the eyes of its owners, of marking the furniture with urine. The kitchen surfaces were wiped down every day, and the cat could never rediscover its markings, so it was not illogical that it should deposit other, less pleasant markers. Little by little, we learned that there was a close correlation between facial pheromonal marking and much more anxiety-inducing urinary marking. Anxious urinary marking makes an appearance when 70 percent of facial marks have been removed. So, if your cat has started urinary marking (as we saw earlier), that means that it hasn't been laying down facial marks for quite some time.

The only time that a cat rubs its cheek on a place and then returns to leave a urinary trace is when it involves sexual marking, and in this case the pheromone in question is F2. But if a cat marks its environment with F3, this prevents urinary marking, and it is on this principle that we vets use synthetic analog diffusers of F3 of the cat's facial pheromone complex. The first such diffuser appeared in 1996, and today we have no fewer than three products that all contain the same synthetic analog of this pheromone.

That leaves just F4. This too has a positive function of recognition, but it is laid on other individuals: this is allomarking, or the marking of others. Yes, you read that correctly: when your cat rubs against you it is a sign, if not of love, then at least of recognition of a positive relationship from which your cat has nothing to fear. Then, anything is possible. It's up to you to construct the rituals and the encounters that will turn this declaration of peace into a declaration of love.

Other Marking Systems

Scratches also have a precise meaning: in the natural environment they indicate the zone of isolation. Most often vertical, they combine a visual signal (stripes) with an olfactory, pheromonal signal: the cat lays down space-marking pheromones via its interdigital sweat glands to indicate that this place is reserved for it alone.

Even in an enclosed space, even in a city apartment, it is not unusual for a cat to scratch next to its main resting place. If this is the bed, then the scratches are often made on the underside and so don't bother anyone. When the cat chooses the sofa as its main zone of isolation, the owners tend to be much less tolerant of the message and can sometimes crack down on it. A punished cat becomes more anxious, which can lead to further scratching or, even worse, incidents of urinary marking. This erodes the relationship even more, the cat is again punished, scolded, or threatened, and a vicious circle ensues.

This is a key message that bears constant repetition: physical sanctions, punishments (that is, anything that inflicts hurt or fear) should be forbidden for cats. They never solve the problem and very often make it worse.

Urinary marking is the final specific marking that my veterinary practice investigates in cats. In our consultations we consider such marking, its recurrence and degree, and build up a behavioral and emotional profile of the cat.

Urinary marking, following a precise sequence, can be reactional. As the term suggests, in these cases it does not indicate a pathological state but rather a dynamic reaction to, for instance, a new object in the house. Let us take the classic example of the sports bag and shoes of the friend who doesn't live in the apartment but drops in now and then on the way back from the gym. Now that you have some grasp of how cats function, you can foresee the different scenarios that might ensue. If we are dealing with a well-balanced cat in a place that it has been able to organize in a way that suits it, then probably a facial marking will be enough to lay down the F3 that will render the object inoffensive. On the other hand, if, for reasons to do with the cat (a more unstable emotional state), the milieu (less well organized), or the object itself (stronger-smelling), facial marking is not enough, urinary marking may occur. Once again, if it is a rare event and only occurs under specific, explicable circumstances, it does not indicate the onset of a pathology. But when this behavior occurs after the cat has stopped facially marking altogether, this should raise a red flag.

Urinary marking involves odors that are familiar to the cat but also alarm pheromones that potential intruders will find off-putting but that can also rebound on the emitter, whose emotional state can get worse if it happens to sniff them. To say "sniff" is not quite accurate: we have considered the physiology of how pheromones are produced, but have not yet devoted any time to how they are detected. There is a specific organ, the vomeronasal or Jacobson's organ, that is dedicated to the perception of these substances. It is linked to the limbic system, hence to the seat of emotions, by the secondary olfactory system. The pheromones are likely to induce an emotional state (calm if it is F3 or F4; troubled if they are alarm pheromones; tender and caring if they are pheromones of adoption) without passing via the cortical filter, thus without consciously registering in the mind of the receiver. This is why pheromones have such a sulfurous reputation: they can induce behavior without the individual's knowledge.

It's worth remembering that if this is the case for insects (from what we know currently), for mammals, and, by definition, for humans, the brain is in charge and will censor undesirable actions. It is a matter of some controversy whether humans of adult age have a vomeronasal organ, though these days it seems to be accepted with certain fundamental differences, including the lack of a secondary olfactory bulb.[13] According to some studies, only 6 percent of us retain a Jacobson's organ as we get older. In some people taste cells take up the role and are capable of detecting pheromones, which can exert their effect.

If you have ever observed your cat, you will no doubt have noticed it make this particular movement: mouth open, eyes narrowed and the tongue making a slight vertical motion. This is called the *flehmen*. Horses do it a lot more spectacularly by rolling up their upper lip, and when male dogs click their tongues while sniffing the urine of a female in heat, it is also the same mechanism. In cats, this discreet movement sends air into the incisor papilla located just behind the dental arch at the incisors, which leads to the Jacobson's organ.

In the case of urinary marking, then, the pheromones contained are alarm pheromones, which are uniquely interspecies and can put dogs as well as cats, and even humans too, on alert. When an animal expresses from its anal glands, which are rich in alarm pheromones, even if the place is cleaned quickly and thoroughly, there are often undetectable pheromones that remain, changing the atmosphere of consultations without anyone being aware.

Now we know how cats construct their living space, which is not the same as ours or that of our dogs, even if we share the same house. Their world is organized and marked. If that is placed under threat, problems can ensue.

Caramel: A Victim of Lockdown

Like many others, whether cats, dogs, or humans, Caramel did not deal with lockdown well, and he made this known in his own feline manner.

For him, this coincided with the start of a new life in which he could go out much more whenever he wanted. Before, he had to ask permission and wait until a human opened the door for him. Just before lockdown, an electronic cat flap was installed. Such devices can help overcome problems with division of the living space, helping to resolve conflicts between the needs of a cat and those of its owners. The electronic settings can be adjusted to allow only one particular cat to enter a room, for example. To control access to the outside, electronic cat flaps do what many parents of teenagers wish they could do: it is possible to allow the cat to come and go as it pleases, but also to program the flap so that the cat can get back in at any time, but can't go out again after eleven o'clock at night, for example.

Caramel was brought in for a consultation because of cleanliness issues. He was eight years old when he came to see me, and these episodes had begun about a year before, right at the beginning of the first lockdown. Christine and Alain also brought along their five-year-old son, Jean. They had moved to a new house when the cat was three and a half.

Upon examining the sequence of events, it became clear that this must be a case of urinary marking, especially since his human companions had tried moving his zone of disposal outdoors, which, now that Caramel had much freer access to the outside, he accepted without difficulty. The litter box was no longer needed: before, it had been well used, and uncleanliness only occurred when it hadn't been cleaned properly; on those occasions, Caramel would defecate right next to the box.

No, what was being described here was a case of urinary marking. Christine often saw him perform the same sequence outside, where it wasn't a problem, and inside, where she and her husband might catch him in the act or come across dried traces after he had been marking. Aside from the inconvenience of the soiling in their house, they were concerned that they never saw him again in normal disposal position but always in marking position. To a vet, this can suggest pollakiuria—that is, the frequent desire to urinate in small quantities, a symptom often associated with certain urinary infections such as cystitis.

Whether a behavioral veterinary doctor or psychiatrist, one always bears in mind, in cats even more than in dogs, how organic illness and behavioral disorders are interconnected. Even before he came to see me, Caramel had had a medical consultation and a urine test, which allowed me to rule out any organic hypothesis, and so the investigation continued. Recalling that, for a cat, micturition is a moment of vulnerability that takes place in a protected space, whereas marking is a form of communication that should be visible and audible, this explained why Caramel's owners never witnessed disposal and saw only marking. But this only got us so far.

Why did an eight-year-old cat suddenly start marking in an increasingly intense and unbridled way? Shopping bags were targeted, but also pullovers or coats that were left on the backs of chairs. One visitor was marked on his trouser leg, and Christine had the unpleasant surprise of receiving a smelly jet from her cat full in the face. Did it have to do with the relationships in the household? Caramel was very friendly with all the humans in the house, including the little boy, with whom he played even though, according to his owners, play was not the cat's favorite activity. If the boy dangled a lure at the end of a toy fishing rod, Caramel would be interested for a few minutes, and the same applied to a laser toy. He was affectionate with his two owners, and it was during a session of cuddling that he sprayed Christine in the face. They were on the sofa at the time, one of his favorite targets.

What made Caramel a complex and interesting case was his apparent lack of consistency. When asked whether he facially marked inanimate objects, Alain and Christine answered in a chorus that he did that a lot. But there was only one place that he scratched: the cat tree next to his sleeping place. Lots of facial and urinary marking but an unchanged pattern of scratching is something one typically sees only in the context of increasing anxiety or with sexual marking. Caramel had been neutered a long time earlier, and it had been more than a year since the marking had begun.

Several elements could have played a part in the onset of an anxious state: there were a host of good reasons for him becoming unsettled in his living space. He had originally lived in an apartment with very restricted access to the outside. Then the child was born, a major disruption in the cat's day-to-day management of its living space. Some pieces of furniture became forbidden or highly monitored, and access was modified. As well as the arrival of an unknown and often noisy newcomer, it is mainly the rearrangement of the space that upsets cats when a newborn joins the household. Then having to stay indoors, but also with the requirement to ask to be let out. And at the same time, he was given great freedom to go out while the humans were obliged to isolate.

I could sense that we were on the right track.

"Do you ever see Caramel with other cats outside?"

"To begin with, there were lots, but Caramel seemed to want to chase them away. We would hear him hissing but we never saw them fight."

"And how was it during the lockdowns?"

"We both—in fact, all three of us—ended up working online," Christine replied with a smile. "So all at once he had more time to spend with Jean, his playmate."

You can see how complex cats are and how much we should avoid projecting our own arrangements and desires onto them. I'm sure Christine was right, and that the cat enjoyed playing more with her boy. I also think he liked being able to explore, discover, and mark out a new outdoor territory, but none of this adaptation was straightforward for a cat who, while not old, was no longer in the first flush of youth.

The base of Maslow's pyramid, the balance of Caramel's living space and his ability to organize it, had been upset by this double challenge: the need to carve out a new outside territory in an area already occupied by other cats, and a part of his indoor territory invaded by humans who normally just passed through at regular times of the day, leaving predictable stretches of time in which the cat could enjoy peace and solitude. It seemed strange to me that the cat had continued to facially mark objects, and I wasn't surprised to receive a message from Alain a few days later saying: "We checked: in fact, Caramel isn't rubbing his head on walls. He sometimes makes the movement, arching his back, but he doesn't seem to leave a trace."

Now it all made sense. All the signs pointed to an anxious state that had been in place for more than a year.

Biotope Repair

My diagnosis of Caramel's behavioral issue was a form of what we vets call *biotopathy*, suffering connected to the biotope or living space. We have already discussed aploutobiotopathy, in which the impoverishment of a cat's territory can reawaken its predatory nature. Here, conversely, we are talking about an environment that had changed a great deal, becoming richer and more complicated. This is *neobiotopathy*, suffering connected to newness in a cat's environment. This could be from new people, rearrangement of furniture, or even a change of rhythm such as that brought about by the pandemic routine. The major symptom of neobiotopathy is more frequent urinary marking.

In a case like this choosing a psychotropic is not too difficult. A hypervigilant cat whose main symptom is urinary marking requires a noradrenergic treatment (which acts on noradrenaline, one of the main neurotransmitters in the brain), and we prescribed clomipramine to Caramel. As we had already tried pheromone diffusers to little avail, we replaced them with aromatherapy diffusers to produce a calming effect on the cat, our patient, but also all the other members of the household. Less easy was finding the right behavioral therapy: understanding what to act upon, what would make sense in this case.

One element of this was straightforward, and we got Christine and Alain on board very quickly: the punishments had to stop. They admitted that in the beginning they had scolded the cat and shown him the traces he made with his marking, but they soon realized this was useless and had read that this could in fact make it worse. We decided to leave periods without any interaction with Caramel when everyone was at home. As for the outside, that was even more difficult, but we found a way forward. When Caramel went out less freely and less frequently, he wasn't marking. While being able to live outside is good for the species in general, it is sometimes worrying, even anxiety-inducing, for a cat who has to face a number of dangers. So reducing Caramel's nighttime excursions was adopted as a protective measure rather than a curtailment of freedom. The only other thing required was a lot of patience.

Understanding the Meaning of Marking

When we take on a case at my clinic, we ask for a report on the cat's marking so we can assess how this might eventually be reduced. When it involves a long-running saga or a chronic condition, the owners are often weary and somewhat impervious to signs of progress. By measuring and quantifying we can get them to stick to it, which buys us the time we need to be able to ameliorate the problem.

Today, Caramel is on course. From two or three episodes of marking a day he is now down to less than one a week: it's still too many, but he is on the road to recovery after three months of treatment. He seems calmer and more back in control of his environment, and now we are no longer in lockdown.

Caramel doesn't want to possess his environment, he just wants to feel good in it, protected, with social encounters alongside stretches of solitude. Together with Alain, Christine, and Jean, I am trying to give him what he wishes.

* * *

Cats' feelings of harmony with their environment are a fundamental key in understanding the feline species. We spend a lot of time putting ourselves in their place to check that their various zones are well located and respected, that their particular and sometimes contradictory needs are satisfied. We should remember that cats are not suburban homeowners.

3

To Relate or Not to Relate

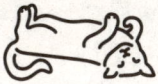

When a cat puts his trust in a man, it is his greatest offering.

—*Charles Darwin*

Cats are companionable animals. At least, that is how they are classified in veterinary medicine. The millions of happy joint histories between cats and the humans who accompany them tend to back this up. Today, the debate around the nature of the relations between humans and their cats can be fraught, however.

For me it seems simple. Cats develop through attachment, just like dogs and just like us humans, but also like lots of other animals—from dolphins, monkeys, elephants, and goats to parrots. In every species, the process of attachment that links the infant to its mother is built via a neuronal, hormonal, and cerebral network that remains active throughout the animal's life and enables individuals to form bonds according to the behavioral repertoire of their species. These range from forming a stable couple to befriending individuals from one's own species or another, whether humans or other animals. This has nothing to do with sociability, which is defined by living in a group with rules, laws, codes, and hierarchies. The relationship that is formed is a dual one, between two individuals, who can be from the same species (though in the case of cats that isn't always the easiest of bonds), or with a suitable individual from another species, particularly one who plays the role of protector, playmate, or provider of care. We don't need a complicated theory to explain their relationships or the problems that they can set off.

If we think of the mother–infant pair as providing the basis for social relations, then in that sense the cat is a social species, but this formulation leaves a lot to be desired. When the relationship is obligatory and asymmetrical, as in a maternal one, there is no need for any apprenticeship; it is innate, and many species display the same sequences. Social relations, on the other hand, rely on learning codes that are different from one species to the next and even among different groups within the same species.

To understand cats' relationships with other living creatures we have to remember they are a nonsocial species. Being both prey and predator, they are born and brought up in a form of attachment the mechanisms of which persist until adulthood and inform strong relationships.

We must dig deeper into this intraspecies relationship—of each cat with other cats—to understand why at the end of the day it can be more complicated than that with individuals of other species. Revisiting a few fundamental points in feline behavior should help us to unravel this.

Tabatha: A Magician without a Wand

Tabatha is a Ragdoll cat, so named because the breed tends to become limp as a rag doll when they are carried, which is not the case with all cats, or all rag dolls for that matter. It is worth reiterating that it is counterfactual, scientifically speaking, to define a whole breed in terms of a particular behavior—a risk for future owners and for the cats. Certain tendencies may be reinforced by lovers of that specific breed, but the fact of belonging to a particular breed cannot be used to predict the behavior of a specific cat. In more scientific terms, the variation within a breed is always greater than the differences between the variant averages of two separate breeds.

Ragdolls have a reputation for being very sociable with dogs, children, and other cats. And they are big: males of the breed can weigh more than twenty pounds. Tabatha weighed twelve pounds and was brought in to us because of cleanliness issues. She lived with Chloé and Alain, as well as Rêveuse, a Chihuahua, with whom she often played. When we checked all the elements that made up her territory, as outlined in the previous chapter, a complex therapeutic picture emerged. The cat displayed both inappropriate disposal behavior on the living-room sofa, where she would be seen squatting, and also clear urinary marking on vertical surfaces and stress-related micturition: on being scolded on one occasion, she even peed out of fear on Alain's knee. Quickly realizing that sanctions were useless, Tabatha's owners stopped all forms of punishment, which put an end to the urination problem but failed to have any effect on the marking and disposals in inappropriate locations.

On the other hand, Tabatha's living space seemed harmonious and her different zones were respected. The marking of inanimate objects hadn't ceased, nor that of living beings, which was significant, and there was still a small amount of scratching. Only the urinary marking and disposal on the bed or the sofa pointed to a pathological state. Moreover, the initial marking was set off by the onset of "flushes," the preliminary phase of estrus—what some describe as a cat being in heat—a typical cause: sexual marking is a classic form of communication in most species.

Subsequently, the cat was spayed, which in theory should resolve all the problems pertaining to sexual marking. But Tabatha's continued.

At the clinic, we pursued our investigation, patiently and in minute detail. When one examines the life of an animal so meticulously, that of a cat in this case, one nearly always discovers ways in which it can be improved. In the case of Tabatha, we advised measures for adjusting her zone of disposal, her litter box, so that it aligned more with ideal criteria. We also noted her preference for wet food, which had led her to reject the kibble that was offered to her. As a result, her meals were probably not frequent enough. I have already highlighted this: a cat, which feeds on small prey and can't devote a lot of time to eating and digesting, will, where possible, snack on between twelve and fifteen small meals a day. As we saw with Coquin in the previous chapter, sometimes it is enough simply to regularize the distribution of food to resolve a behavioral issue. But at the clinic we sensed that this wasn't the case with Tabatha.

A consultation is a search, a sort of treasure hunt, and sometimes one finds the answer through a flash of inspiration, a sudden revelation. All at once, the root of the problem is clear. This was a loving cat and she couldn't bear to be separated from her human companions. Tabatha suffered from anxious attachment that wasn't properly addressed.

The mist dispersed, bit by bit.

"Is Tabatha aggressive?"

"Never! Quite the opposite!"

"What do you mean by 'quite the opposite'?"

"We sometimes feel like we have a dog: Tabatha follows us around, greets us when we come home."

"And where does she rest?"

"In the evening, when we are both sitting on the sofa, she often comes and lies between us."

"Does she do that when she sleeps too?"

"Yes, she sometimes sleeps between us," Chloé confirmed.

And Alain added with a smile, and a nod toward his wife: "But it's not her favorite place. What she really likes is sleeping in Chloé's arms."

This extreme sharing of the resting place, the zone of isolation, leads one to seek signs of suffering caused by separation.

In this cat, they were subtle but constant. The couple remembered going on a trip for a few days and leaving the cat in the good hands of a friend. She fed her, spent time with her, and everything seemed to be going fine. However, they found, on their return, that Tabatha had lost the fur between her ears and on her face between the eyes. She wasn't bald, but the fur was much thinner, a sign that she had been scratching or overzealous in her facial marking. We now know that this can become more frequent at the start of an anxious state. Without her usual humans around her, one can imagine that Tabatha had difficulty maintaining her emotional equilibrium, hence increasing her facial marking, though this had not been enough.

Missing You Already

If an adult animal cannot find the right balance emotionally when the subject of its attachment goes away, its suffering is connected to a lack of autonomy. The ability to maintain sensory homeostasis in the absence of members of the group is one of the markers of adulthood. In social species, such as dogs or human beings, there are a number of hacks for managing social distance. We sometimes need to separate ourselves from our loved ones and then find them again. Online happy hours organized during the pandemic were an expression of this inescapable necessity. For nonsocial animals such as cats, it is not a species necessity, but it can be an individual need.

These days, we call this behavioral disorder marked by the inability to maintain equilibrium in the absence of the subject of attachment *autonomopathy*:[1] a term we use to indicate that the suffering (*-pathy*) is connected to the absence of autonomy. This condition has long been known as *separation anxiety*. Indeed, the first international publication to suggest that some behavioral problems in cats might relate to separation used this term in its title.[2] We chose to stop using this term for cats and dogs in France both to avoid confusion with human medicine and to be more clear and precise. Not all animals who suffer from autonomopathy are in an anxious state: some may be in a phobic state, some may be anxious, and others depressive. Establishing the cause, the etiology, need not entail identifying a pathological state: that is one of the main reasons why we changed the name.

For Tabatha, then, we needed to increase her level of autonomy, which normally does not pose a problem for cats. I would be prepared to wager that we will see more and more of these cases, since changing lifestyles and shifts in our understanding of cats can be disruptive to their behavioral balance. For a long time, except among a few artists and eccentrics, the cat was merely a weapon in the human battle against vermin, but now our view has completely changed. Today, cats are welcomed into the heart of our homes, and all we ask from them is their company, which is actually a big ask in feline terms and may even prove too much for them.

If we take a historical view, we may ask ourselves whether this hasn't in fact been the case for quite some time: archaeology is always very illuminating. Where did the cat buried in the tomb of a rich Cypriot around 9500 BC and discovered in 2004 at the Shillourokambos site on Cyprus by Jean-Denis Vigne and his team of archaeologists come from?[3] Cats are not native to the island, and it is too far from the nearest mainland for them to have gotten there under their own steam. It must have been the island's first colonizers who brought the feline with them; even though it may not have been of any practical use, it clearly had a great value.

What may have been an eccentricity at the time has become the norm, and we now recognize in cats such a propensity for attachment that, as we have already seen, in France they have become by far our principal animal companion.

And There's the Cure

Tabatha needed her creatures of attachment, which is normal, but she couldn't bear their prolonged absence, which is a sign of pathology. To recalibrate the attachment so that it no longer generated stress, my colleagues and I put in place what we called a "meeting therapy": Tabatha's "parents" would refuse her demands for contact, but several times a day they would offer her some moments of cuddling or interaction.

At first the treatment didn't progress smoothly. For a while, denial of contact aggravated the symptoms. This is par for the course in therapy. At that point we were relying on an anti-anxiety medical treatment, put in place to help us get through the worst of it. It worked well with Tabatha after six weeks: she was calmer, happy again, and clean. She unfailingly urinated only in her litter boxes, which were kept spotless and placed in the optimal locations. If you think that that should have been enough and it was unnecessary to go looking for complicated causes or explain it with funny-sounding medical terms, Tabatha herself provided confirmation of the root of the problem when she relapsed the first time her human companions went away for a few days.

Cats are not hardwired to live in human society, but rather are nourished by attachment and can form passionate relationships sometimes to an excessive degree, and to the point of pathology when absence causes suffering. Today, Tabatha is doing much better, but we are aware that she still suffers from a potential emotional imbalance, and each absence has to be carefully managed from an environmental, behavioral, and biological point of view. There is a good chance, now that she no longer suffers from anxiety, that nutritional supplements might prevent her from relapsing when she is left alone for a few days.

Vets have been noticing that more cats are very attached (that is still okay!) or even hyperattached, and in the latter case it takes little more than their owners being absent for the weekend to tip them into pathology. It is worth noting that it was because Tabatha presented undesirable behaviors such as soiling that her owners sought help. So we were able to discover her anxious state, dig down to the root of it, and treat the whole problem. But what would have happened if her anxiety had been less apparent, and her main symptom had just been excessive licking rather than undesirable disposals?

Perhaps nothing. Many cats suffer because they exhibit so little, which means no one can understand their suffering.

One of the major points in feline behavioral psychology, apart from problems connected to territory (biotopathies), which we have already discussed, is the difficulty of maintaining sometimes challenging relationships. This all springs from the lack of a social structure in the feline world. Sociopathic tendencies have been identified in dogs,[4] but there is a difference between cases of human and canine sociopathy. The former arise from psychosis, while the latter are connected to the occasional difficulty of establishing clear and reassuring rules in an interspecies group. In both cases, this relates to a species that lives in a social group, establishing codes and obeying rules, which is easier for certain individuals to accept than others.

None of this applies to the cat: no hierarchies, no social group. Cats do, however, have one-to-one relationships that bring them reassurance and pleasure but that, conversely, may also cause problems and, in more serious cases, anxiety or depression. Before we get to these pathological states, let us first turn to "bottle kittens," meaning kittens found without a mother and bottle-fed, which can lead to very complicated developmental issues.

Luka: Into the Wild

Luka was one of those cases that the pandemic brought in, characteristic of both the deep ethological roots of our domestic feline and its change of status, but also the way in which vets are now paying attention to behavioral pathology. Aware of the abnormality and the urgency of the situation, his vet did not hesitate to refer this two-month-old kitten to my clinic.

When I saw Luka he was only two months and fourteen days old, smashing the record for the youngest cat I'd treated in my time as a specialist in cat behavior. I have a certain fondness for this cat and his humans, Lydie and Rémi. Not so very long ago, this cat would have been abandoned, dumped in the street where he was found, put down, or perhaps kept with considerable danger to the owners. But here everyone was striving to preserve the relationship, to maintain the bond by caring for this little cat through all the means at our disposal with due regard for his physical health and his well-being.

Luka's story was quite moving: in the deserted streets of the umpteenth lockdown, Lydie heard a plaintive meowing. When she looked, she found three newborn kittens: she didn't touch them or take them with her, assuming quite reasonably that the mother might come back to find them. To set her mind at rest, she kept an eye on them for the rest of the day to see if they were actually picked up. When night fell, with freezing temperatures forecast, Lydie decided to go fetch the kittens and take care of them, since she was sure that they would not survive the cold. She took them home, but two of the three kittens died that night: only Luka survived.

Lydie and Rémi took care of him after seeking advice from their vet: they fed him with good-quality baby milk, showered him with affection, and were quite baffled when, as he developed his psychomotor abilities, Luka showed increasingly aggressive behavior, often inflicting wounds on them when they had contact with him. Like every "parent," like every person in an educating role, Lydie and Rémi thought they must have gotten something wrong and so felt largely responsible for Luka's problems.

And now I had the little devil before me. There seemed to be a wild energy coursing through his tiny body. During the consultation, he played with everything that he could get his paws on: the sheet of paper on the bench, the slats of the blinds when he brushed against them or hid behind them. During my consultations, I interact a lot with my patients, and, while I am a proponent of telemedicine as an additional resource, there is no doubt that direct contact with a patient is both valuable in gaining information and a constant source of pleasure. With Luka, the pleasure had a sharp edge to it. I noticed a number of things when I started playing with him: he wasn't afraid of me, or the interaction, or the environment. He was very active, even more reactive, and he could not tolerate any constraint. Whenever I prevented him from moving, his ears would flatten and he would take a swipe with claws out at anything within reach.

The funniest—but also very significant—moment of the consultation was undoubtedly when he seemed to mistake Rémi for a tree, climbing onto his shoulders, then onto his head, before starting to "attack" his ears, which didn't move a millimeter. After filming it for educational purposes, we interrupted Luka, who didn't take kindly to being removed from his latest plaything.

No Limits

To explain what this cat was suffering from, let us revisit a few things we have learned: like Nougat, Luka had not acquired the correct mechanisms of self-control, but where for Nougat and his fellow sufferers from HSHA that was the sole root of the problem, Luka was also unable to inhibit himself, which is a prerequisite for any successful relationship. We are not talking here about submission or hierarchy, which are the preserve of social species, but inhibition, the ability to restrain certain reactions in order to establish contact with another living being. We have seen in different contexts how Nougat, with his lack of self-control mechanisms, and Lucifer, whose anxious state triggered harmful attacks, could also jeopardize the relationship with their owners, but at least they were able to build one in the first place.

Luka was not able to do so. Having had no contact with his mother, despite the goodwill and attention his owners had devoted to his development, he lacked tolerance and constraint.

In the new terminology of feline behavioral pathology, my colleagues and I wanted to focus in particular on relationships, and so we coined the term *schezipathy*. The Greek root combines *schezi-*, relation, and *-pathy*, suffering. Unlike humans and dogs, cats cannot be sociopathic but instead have schezipathies. It's not the social relation, with its roster of rules, that is the cause of the problem but the simple relationship between two individuals. While this does not involve any hierarchy, it inevitably requires self-inhibition, the acceptance of certain constraints and the ability to synchronize with the other.

Not all types of relationships are suitable for certain cats—as we will see later—and some cats are not prepared for relationships because of developmental problems. Those like Luka who are incapable of the slightest inhibition suffer from *aschezia*. The name of this condition, indicating an absence of any relationship, should not be taken literally, however: it is neither a condemnation nor a gloomy prognosis. It merely states where we are starting from. If they are deprived of maternal contact and guidance in self-control, kittens do not have a user's manual when it comes to relations between two individuals. For years vets thought that these kittens were not good candidates for adoption, but the work of Joëlle Hofmans on interdisciplinary behavioral veterinary medicine has shown that the opposite is in fact the case.[5]

To differentiate kittens detached prematurely from their mother from those who have benefited from a longer apprenticeship with the mother cat, we test their carrying reflex (being lifted by the scruff of the neck—note, it's not violent and is definitely not a punishment—see box). If the kitten adopts a fetal or relaxed position, this indicates that it has been in contact with its mother for up to eight weeks or longer. On the other hand, if it goes into a state of hyperextension, threatening, with its claws out, this tends to suggest that it has not had the benefit of maternal contact beyond five weeks. The thinking behind this is that kittens with a "poor" carrying reflex make less companionable cats than those who have had a demonstrably more harmonious upbringing. But the results showed the opposite. People who acquired a cat with a poor carrying reflex declared themselves more satisfied after a year than those who had acquired a cat that had been raised normally.

Testing the Carrying Reflex Is Not a Form of Punishment

Grabbing a cat by the scruff of the neck is a diagnostic test; it reproduces a standard maneuver of the mother when she changes the nest site and covers her tracks to escape would-be predators. It is in no way a punishment.

I often hear clients say this when I raise the issue of punishments or physical sanctions in the case of uncleanliness, for example. When they understand that they are not being judged but rather listened to, many tell me that at times, when they have felt exasperated by finding their bed once again stained with urine, they have taken the cat by the scruff of the neck and shaken it with a certain degree of force to "explain to it that it shouldn't do that; that it's wrong." Now that you are better informed about cat behavior, you will know that this can never work. Either the reflex is still active, and there will be a disconnect between the small feline and its environment, or it isn't, in which case the punishment will be painful and will trigger an aggressive response. But in neither case will the cat learn anything.

My colleagues and I had to think about what this meant, and we noticed that the kittens with the poor reflex, as anticipated, showed many more signs of anxiety, and their usual way of dealing with this was to develop an exaggerated attachment to their human. For example, they spent much more time on their owner's lap than the "normal" kittens, which, in their first year, spend much more time playing, cavorting, exploring, than looking for cuddles. So they suffered from a behavioral disorder, but they learned their resilience from the bond with their owner, who then felt invested. Attachment was still at the root of this paradox, but we were forced to revise our original judgment.

Not all cats who have a poor carrying reflex are aschezic. While it can often be an element that leads us to suspect this condition, it is important to emphasize that things can improve. It was some volunteers from a cat rescue charity who taught me not to be too categorical in my prognosis. When I saw cats that I never thought would become sociable change their attitude and become very familiar and friendly, sometimes with a single person, but often with all humans, I had to accept that a bad start in life did not predetermine everything. Especially nowadays, when the treatments that are available enable us to reduce the danger and prolong cohabitation.

Not a Good Start

Luka is a living example of this paradox. When I tested his carrying reflex, I expected a strong reaction on his part, and sure enough, he began hissing and struggling, but, after a few seconds, I felt him suddenly relax in my hand and in the end it was more like the positive reflex of a kitten who has had a normal development.

That told me that this kitten was already on the way to being healed, even if at the time of the consultation his life was still difficult for him. To repeat our mantra: physical punishment is never suitable for cats. It never resolves problems and aggravates anxiety. The mistake comes from the fact that—and there is plenty of room for discussion here—it might be considered an effective sanction in a puppy provided it is applied moderately, simultaneously, and carried out in the way a puppy's mother would do it—that is, by pressing the puppy to the ground by the scruff of the neck. None of this applies with cats. Although their mothers spend a lot of time educating them and controlling them, they never use this method.

Luka received two or three small taps from his humans (something that feline mothers might do), which were not hard, and disruptive rather than punitive, but it didn't have any effect. So Rémi, the main target of the violent games, would scold and threaten the cat but without ever striking him. Analysis of the subsequent behavioral signs confirmed improvement after a very difficult start. Luka had been voracious when he took the bottle: he got annoyed, let go of it, then took it again like a child with an insatiable hunger, frustrated that he could never feel full. He then regulated himself, having been refused permission to come to the table (these very lively little cats often pounce on the plates to pilfer food), without force but firmly, while at the same time being offered constant access to a bowl of top-quality cat kibble.

Teaching cleanliness came early: Lydie had read up on it and received some good advice. Having had the kitten for only one or two days, at the time when his sphincters weren't yet functioning, she knew that it was necessary to mimic the behavior of the mother cat to activate the perineal reflex. A gentle massage of the lower belly and the perineal zone was enough to trigger excretion, and it was then possible to wipe the kitten with toilet paper or a soft paper towel. Keeping a kitten alive at the start of its life is all well and good, but it is so much better if you can also teach it the key points of how it should function. Lydie knew this and she demonstrated the use of the litter box to Luka by scratching and depositing some of his stools and then covering them up. Like a kitten being guided by its mother, Luka was clean within four weeks.

His marking behavior was somewhat out of kilter: he had never done any urinary marking, nor any facial marking on inanimate objects (or at least not yet; he was ten weeks old when I first saw him). He rubbed against his owners a lot, a bit too much for their liking, and I agreed, as it all ended in out-of-control games and harmful attacks.

As for his disposal regime, even though it had been established quite early on, it included a few bizarre habits. After a few weeks of treatment, when the attacks had mostly been brought under control, Luka would select the top of the litter box as his resting place. Like many young couples, Lydie and Rémi didn't have a big apartment and had opted for a litter box with a lid to hide the feces and minimize the smell. Luka had decided to make it one of his favorite zones of isolation. We tried to redirect him to other places that were more suitable by enticing him with food or games, but Luka seemed impervious to these suggestions.

What happened with our little devil, who had been deprived of maternal control and education but had evolved more or less normally thanks to the careful attention of his humans? As he reinvented his behavioral repertoire as one of an (almost) normal cat, Luka began to seek zones of isolation that were more protected. I suggested to Lydie that she buy one of those furry "igloos." Like a very cozy little tent, they cater to a cat's dual need to be protected and to be able to see without being seen. After some initial hesitation, Luka adopted his new cabin and abandoned his litter box except when using it for its proper function.

It's Not All Set in Stone from Birth

Luka's story seems to me an exemplary one, but let's not count our chickens. This story helps us answer a crucial question in our discipline: Does everything get played out in early development or is it at all possible to alter the course of destiny?

I am fully aware that many couples in Lydie and Rémi's position would have given up and kicked Luka out into the street, but my feeling is that more and more cat owners are trying to strike a better balance between their everyday lives and the well-being of their animals. Our role as vets is to protect that relationship, to understand the fears and exasperations of the humans, to be familiar with the fundamental needs of each species that we care for but even more to be able to decode what each individual animal needs to achieve balance.

Psychiatry—both human and veterinary—is often criticized on two scores. First, everything is seen in terms of psychopathology, which runs the risk of no longer considering any behavior as normal, or on the contrary of no longer being able to define the limits of what is acceptable. And second, it is prescriptive, based on the definition of health provided by the World Health Organization in 1946, which has never been questioned since: "Health is a state of complete physical, mental, and social well-being and not merely the absence of disease or infirmity."[6]

Including social well-being was very controversial. If someone is dissatisfied with the society in which they live, should this be defined as an illness? I think we all know the answer to this question. The danger is obvious: "treating" someone for social illness implies a form of psychiatry weaponized as enforced social harmony. In the vast majority of cases, it is quite the opposite, and psychiatrists are attentive, tolerant, and understanding in a way that is inspiring and deserving of respect.

Cats Do Not Have Social Norms

Dogs and cats have no need to adhere to social norms. This is debatable in the case of dogs, which are not supposed to be a nuisance and which sometimes find themselves in the spotlight when they are "dangerous." And what about cats? They do not occupy any social space—except for stray cats, which the authorities have to deal with—and so are not expected to conform to any social norm. So the veterinary psychiatrist does not want to impose normativity and intervenes only for the good of their health, their emotional balance, and their well-being. For us vets, tracing the dividing line between the normal and the pathological is our bread and butter.

The definition of normality is also a matter of culture, place, and time and, for a species, whether or not it is domesticated.

Domesticated or Tamed?

I was struck by the fact that, despite the discovery of other cat graves on Cyprus (indicating that the animals were loved), Jean-Denis Vigne and his colleagues said that they preferred not to use the word "domestication" in the case of cats, and the aforementioned feline found at the Shillourokambos site was a large animal, a wildcat.[7] The scientists preferred to use the word "taming" (the term "domestication" being used more rarely). Nowadays, the question of how exactly we understand our cats informs the discussion around support for their behavioral disorders. Are we talking about a domesticated animal, or rather a liminal animal who shares our private space but is not yet completely domesticated?

Bear in mind that the very definition of this word is always subject to controversy. The social or the biological aspect may predominate, depending on the author's academic background. Along with the American zooarchaeologist Nerissa Russell,[8] I think that both should be taken into consideration. With the cat, everything depends on what you decide to look at. If we consider only cat breeding, then we are clearly talking about domestication, given alterations in morphology, the creation of hypertypes, and distortions that are then retained as characteristics of the breed, in an environment that only allows reproduction to take place in a very specific, human-led context. But you only need to turn to the charities that take care of street cats to come to the opposite conclusion: the morphology of cats has not changed much in a very long time, and many would like to have better control of their reproduction.

Cat protection organizations tend to brandish scary figures: in four years, a couple of unsterilized cats can be responsible for the birth of more than 20,000 kittens, which makes your head spin, though this has never been put to the test. This theoretical number does not take account of any regulating factors. This explains this modern version of the endlessly leaking tub of the Danaïdes: capturing cats and sterilizing them has never eradicated a population of stray cats. It was decades before large numbers of local government, cat protection, and veterinary staff understood this and set cats free after sterilization, which was made possible by the disappearance of rabies as an endemic disease in France. It is much more effective to capture cats, spay or neuter them, and then release them to their normal living space than to eliminate them. Nature abhors a void, and if there are corners of the world that are congenial to cats, you will find cats there, whether you like it or not. Hopefully those that have been spayed or neutered, who will not contribute to population explosion.

So, are cats domesticated? Not entirely. Most of our domestic cats could revert to the wild and be self-sufficient, feeding off small prey. Even today it sometimes happens that cats return to a life without contact with humans and with no assistance from them. If they hang around people's houses feeding off scraps, they are called strays. If they go back to the forests away from human habitation, they are known as feral cats.

We can learn a lot from the existence of these cats: their journey to domestication comes with the option of a return ticket. A species that has had the "good fortune" to live in contact with human beings can decide to liberate itself from them. I think that this is one of the reasons for the ire they arouse, which sees them accused of multiple evils, of which the most serious today is their threat to biodiversity. The feline species dares to spurn the notion that domestic bliss with human beings is an unmissable opportunity.

And what should we psychiatric vets do? Where do we place ourselves on this spectrum between the wild at one end and the domestic at the other?

Care and Concern

The behavioral treatment we offer our patients is—it bears repeating—neither normative nor moralizing. We have scientific evidence to back up the fact that an indoor life can, under certain conditions, be a harmonious one for a cat and that while an outdoor life can sometimes be more stimulating, it also has lots of dangers. What is good for the species is not always good for the individual cat. Far from it.

Our mission as psychiatric vets is therefore clear. We must dispense with the dogmatic view that the idea of a domestic, enclosed cat—a captive cat, as some call them—is somehow intolerable or that a cat must be able to go out in order to express to the full its predator–prey nature, with all the risks that may be entailed. Rather we must approach each case with care and concern: we are there for the cat, attentive to the unique reality of each individual, to the way in which it succeeds or fails in adapting to its environment, according to its resources, and to the consequences of its relationships with the other living creatures in its environment.

In full knowledge of the facts, we have to verify that the five freedoms (or the five needs, or the five areas dear to theorists of well-being) are respected, as well as the five pillars[9] of creating a positive environment for a cat (see box). These feed back into the debate on normality: given a cat's dual nature, I believe there are more ways of being "normal" for a cat than for a dog, and there is no need to file everything away under pathology.

The Five Pillars of a Healthy Environment for a Cat
(According to the International Society for Feline Medicine)

Pillar 1: Provide a safe place.

Pillar 2: Plan separate spaces for different resources: food, water, toilet zone, scratching zone, play zone, and zone of rest or sleep.

Pillar 3: Provide opportunities for play and to exercise predator behavior.

Pillar 4: Offer positive, coherent, and predictable social interactions.

Pillar 5: Make sure the cat's environment respects the importance of its senses and sense of smell in particular.

We also have reliable indicators of suffering, of an inability to adapt, that constitute clear markers of behavioral pathology. So, in the case of Luka, the position seemed clear. This kitten seemed destined for certain death; he was offered a chance to survive, and was carefully looked after. However, the trauma of the first days of his short life, at a critical stage in his development, and his individual vulnerability put him on the road to pathology, which entailed suffering for him and danger for others. Our role as vets was to alleviate this suffering, to equip Luka with new ways of adapting, and to help him recover his self-control and ability to inhibit impulsive responses. Once his medical treatment was completed, we could continue solely with therapy, which would better fit into the life of the family. Let me highlight at this point something that I know concerns a number of my clients: no, we do not envisage treatment being for life. We use medication to restore brain plasticity, and, except in very rare cases, the general rule is to stop administering treatments after a certain period of time—six, twelve, or eighteen months, depending on the case, the diagnosis, the initial prognosis, and the intensity of the therapeutic work carried out in parallel.

Luka was given a psychotropic to control his levels of serotonin—the neurotransmitter involved in lack of control and harmful aggressive behavior, according to our current model.

Help to Develop Self-Control

It's a classic form of therapy, but an effective one: stop all physical sanctions (there weren't that many in Luka's case) and verbal threats. Being afraid can trigger as many phobic responses as being ill in the first place. On the other hand, it is easy in a "normal" kitten to teach, for example, the command "soft paw" by pressing on its toes to make it retract its claws to prevent scratching games from getting out of hand. In Luka's case, the control provided by the medication allowed this instruction to take place. Redirecting the attacks to permitted toys is also sensible, but, at the risk of sounding contrary, I think it is crucial to let the kitten continue to play with your hands so that you can monitor the acquisition of self-control of its claws and teeth. In Luka's case, the nips and cuts became fewer and farther between, and things started to improve. Luka is still making progress; he has relapses from time to time, but they are less severe. Lydie and Rémi handle him with tenderness and respect, and I am savoring this victory.

Luka represents an extreme but revealing case of the difficulty certain "bottle cats" have in developing basic relationships. Such cases are not rare, but it's worth saying it again: cats like this respond to treatment, and though this requires empathy and knowledge, their prognosis is not bad. One of the last videos recorded as part of Luka's follow-up shows a large adult cat lying next to his human and rubbing up against them. The short note that accompanied the video said: "We thought you might like this." And, indeed, I liked it very much.

There are tens, maybe hundreds of thousands of cats who suffer a mismatch between their ability to form relationships and what is expected of them: so many interspecies misunderstandings. It is time to do them justice and restore hope to everyone.

Isis: Into the Depths of Hell

Once again, it's important to reiterate that cats are not dogs. I see so many cases where, not for reasons of malice but rather an inability to think outside the box, cats are treated like dogs.

There are many similarities between the two species: they both belong to the order of carnivores and have lived with humans for thousands of years. They both develop through attachment, and that enables them throughout their adult lives to form positive relationships. They also live in a shared sensory world: their five senses are equally keen, in particular their sense of smell, which is so much more developed than ours, bringing them closer to that world. They are both neotenic species, in which certain juvenile characteristics persist throughout their adult lives, such as the capacity to play. So the confusion is understandable.

Aline and Raymond brought their cat to see me in a large veterinary practice in the Paris region. It was winter, and both of them were wrapped up in thick jackets, which, I would soon discover, didn't just provide protection against the cold. My patient was a small black cat with short hair. She was unworried about leaving her cat carrier and came toward me without hesitation. I stroked her once, but the second time I touched her, she froze and started hissing. This was meant to be threatening, like the way a dog growls. It says: "Keep your distance!" and "Hands off!"

I held off after this introduction and asked why they had come today.

"You've just seen for yourself," Aline replied. "Isis attacks! She frightens me! . . . And on top of all that, she is unclean."

These few words summed up the two most common complaints we hear in feline behavioral medicine: they are the tip of the iceberg.

Isis walked around the consultation room, jumped onto Aline's lap, stepped across onto Raymond, then back to Aline, who stroked her; at the fourth or fifth touch, the threatening behavior began again. I observed Isis: although her carrier was open, she didn't go inside. She walked in front of it a few times, sniffed it but didn't take refuge inside, as most of her fellow cats would have done when deciding not to grace us with their important presence during a consultation.

Each time she walked past, she rubbed the part of her head just below the ear against Aline and Raymond, which led one or the other of them to attempt to touch her. She tolerated the first two or three strokes, but the next one would cause her, at the very least, to turn around, hiss, spit, and often take a more or less forceful swipe with her paw.

Suffering in Resonance

The work of a veterinary psychiatrist is based, on the one hand, on our ever-expanding understanding of the functioning of the brain and of neurotransmitters and their receptors, and, on the other, on empathy, which must be directed both toward the animal whose behavior we are trying to interpret and also toward the humans who accompany our patient. In a case like that of Isis, if we take the strictest sense of the word "patient"—one who suffers—then it is equally applicable to the owners. Even though Isis was officially my patient, I could also see the human suffering involved. There was no question of me taking the place of a psychologist, psychiatrist, or family counselor, but the aspect of the relationship that impacted the animal did come within my scope of intervention. If I could understand in the first instance, then explain, and with the cooperation of my clients provide the solutions to releasing them from this painful vise, then I would have cared for the animal—my primary mission—but also improved the well-being of all concerned.

My work always starts with observing the animal while listening to the narrative presented by the humans who live with it. The human point of view always accompanies what we can establish about the animal's feelings. It is a point of animal ethics that it seems to me important to underline. By definition our pets are heteronomous—subject to the decisions of the humans who accompany them, cherish them, and sometimes mistreat them. Strictly speaking, they can never express their own opinion even if their behavior, their reactions speak for them. We now have the means to assess the suffering and identify the pathological states of our domestic felines, although this does not provide a complete picture of their thoughts and emotions.

Observing Isis provided quite a few clues: She didn't have an aversion to humans, or an excessive fear of being touched. She didn't try to run away from us and in fact was capable of being interested in contact with a stranger. She looked for reassurance by coming up to her humans and practicing allomarking (rubbing to lay down familiarization pheromones) on them, which points to a high-quality attachment. There were clear positive signs in this relationship, but how could it have deteriorated to the point where a pathological state had been precipitated, with clear signs of intermittent anxiety, urinary marking, and irritable aggression?

Having examined the cat's behavior, it was time to find out more about the humans.

"Tell me, when and how did the first attacks occur?"

While we were talking, Isis jumped onto Aline's knee and started rubbing against her chin. I could sense Aline's fear as soon as contact was made.

"Well, a bit like this actually. . . . In the evening Isis would come to me when I was lying down and rub herself against my head, like you just saw. I would stroke her, but one time she suddenly bit me hard on the chin. I gave a yell, and she ran off."

"Did that happen just the once?"

"No. We had this routine of cuddles at bedtime. Every evening she would come and rub herself against me while purring. But on the day after she had bitten me, I was more guarded. I stroked her head a little bit, but when I sensed that she was about to bite me again, I pushed her away."

"Altogether, how many times has this happened?"

"Maybe four or five times? A couple of times at least, when I thought we were in the middle of a lovely cuddle, she bit me on the chin, and I chased her away. And then she started peeing as well!"

"And how did you react?"

"Like we'd been told to. I showed it to her, stuck her nose in it, and then gave her a little tap to let her know it was not okay."

Making headway with clients relies on being nonjudgmental, even if one knows in a case like this that certain responses by the owner might aggravate the situation. We always take account of the fact that they meant well. No blame should be attached to an action if it is made in good faith in the belief that it is the correct response.

Understanding, Not Coercion

For cats relationships are an optional extra. Since they are by definition a nonsocial species, they do not possess mechanisms for collaboration or, especially, reconciliation. And since they are a species with a dual nature, as predator and prey, cats are prone to heightened sensitivity, including in their relationships. This means that if a relationship, even a special one, starts to become frightening or dangerous, the cat can give up on it and react negatively to being touched.

In fact, I'll let you in on a secret: cats keep a little red book in their inside pocket in which they note down any unpleasant events. The notes in this book are never erased. You must at all costs avoid going down in that book, and to that end must have a perpetual ban on punishments or threats.

Even if your cat has just urinated on the curtains for the umpteenth time or broken a precious vase, before giving it a smack or shouting at it, think about that little red book and restrain yourself. This doesn't mean you have to accept everything or that it is impossible to educate a cat, but this never works through coercion. In other words, don't trash the relationship. For Aline and Isis, things had deteriorated badly, but there was a way back.

Bite–Smack: A Bad Combination

Isis loved her human friend, and biting was for her a confusion of love and suffering, a sign of the pleasure of the encounter and the start of a misunderstanding. There were no preceding markers of aggression: the biting reflected excitement, not an assault. We can understand Aline, bitten by surprise when she was expecting a show of tenderness, and her instinctive defensive reaction, but this made no sense to the cat, who was delighting in the affectionate encounter. What followed was mistrust and sensitivity on both sides: for Isis, the human friend had become unpredictable, capable of threatening or smacking—something to be noted on the first page of the little red book. Imagine the cat's confusion: upset by a broken bond, disoriented by this new unpredictability, Isis did what cats do—try to establish harmony by marking her territory, especially through urinary marking, a sign that the situation was going downhill. Subsequent punishments would only exacerbate the situation. What gave us hope was that the biting had begun only a few weeks ago, and the urinary marking even more recently: it was still possible to put things right. Isis had started to express signs of intermittent anxiety, which we would treat, but this would only work if my analysis of the situation could break the vicious circle.

Once again, during the consultation, Isis jumped on the knee of her human companion, who stroked her and then gave her a light pinch of the tail, although this was in fact perceived as a threat. Isis nevertheless came back to rub against Aline's chin as she stroked her, and I called a halt.

"Stop! Just one stroke . . . wait until she asks for more contact. She wants to be on you, against you, maybe even to leave marks of familiarization, but that doesn't mean that she wants to be touched, or that she finds it pleasant."

"But if she comes to me, it must mean she wants to be stroked."

"No, if she comes to you, it's because she wants to sit on you."

Aline looked surprised, and I could understand why.

"When we humans sit on each other's laps, we're generally expecting, or hoping, that something else will happen."

Aline and Raymond both laughed out loud at this, and I smiled with them.

"But for cats, it's not at all obvious. As you have seen: since the start of the consultation, Isis has come to you looking for reassurance, but as soon as you touch her, she leaves again. You are her refuge, but you have to imagine you're wearing gloves of fire. If you stroke her once, that's fine, but if you carry on you will 'burn' her, or at least cause her distress."

Interpreting

I was being an interpreter. The human species and the feline species have different behavioral programs, and misinterpretations can often occur even if, in general, it is not so difficult to strike up a rapport with cats. We boast that we have the most highly developed mental capacities, so let's use them to better understand those who choose to live with us in friendship. As we have seen, with cats that is never written in stone.

This is always a key moment in the consultation: often, the diagnosis is not difficult but, to give the therapy the best chance of working, it is important to build a good therapeutic alliance. The owners of the animal have to share an understanding of the root of the problem. In this case, I could tell that Aline and Raymond were not convinced by my initial explanations, but what I said about laps and gloves of fire changed their minds. Isis helped me here: during the hour-long consultation, she had demonstrated how important they were for her, how much they were her refuge. This was the basis for a reassuring and strong attachment, and I could tell Aline that her cat loved her and there was no need to look for the cause of the problem anywhere else than in this ethological (indeed almost cross-cultural) misinterpretation.

Building a Respectful Relationship

Caring for an animal always involves the practitioner's skill, the willingness of its owners to effect improvement, and, last but not least, the participation of the animal itself. Everyone has to be on board with a common vision. And everyone should be a winner: primarily our patient, the cat, but also the humans who accompany it.

In the case of Isis, no longer being punished and being able to enjoy nonintrusive contact with her human companions were the two main imperatives. Although Aline and Raymond now knew that their cat might want to approach them but not to be touched, they would still like to have more contact. It was Isis who gave me the idea of setting up a therapy of desire.

Obtaining Consent, or the Therapy of Desire

A cat should be able to express its wish to control the quantity of caresses and limit them according to its wishes. You have to establish a contact signal: for example, offer your hand as a closed fist with the middle finger slightly protruding. If the cat rubs against your finger, it's as if it is giving you a ticket for contact. Then apply a gentle, slow, and smooth caress. Finish off with a light touch, but don't pinch the tail, of course. Offer your hand again in the same way, and if the cat rubs again, you can start stroking again—but if it doesn't seek contact, stop there.

After a few such sessions, Isis learned that she wouldn't be touched except when she wanted it. Ceasing punishments reduced her anxiety, assisted by the medication, which was selected to diminish her hypervigilance and curtail her marking behavior. Medication alone would not have sufficed. It has to be connected to an evaluation of the pathological state and the therapy that will restore balance. Psychotropics are often a necessary part of treatment, but are never enough in themselves.

Make a Date with Your Cat

We also prescribe a meeting therapy. If you want a shared moment with your dog, in most cases all you need to do is call it. Yes, yes, I know; you have a cat who always comes when called and is always up for contact. There are exceptions to every rule when it comes to cats. But let's stick with the general rule. Flora, my last feline companion, was an affectionate and gentle cat, provided that she wasn't cooped up. I knew the two places and times when I would be guaranteed a long session of cuddles and purring: the evening, in front of the fireplace, though if the dogs were nearby she wouldn't come; and last thing at night or in the morning in bed, when she loved to sleep on my back or my chest, purring, rubbing against me, and playing Simon's Cat, which was enough to wake her human companion.[10] My rendezvous with another one of my cats, Chiquita, was at seven in the evening on the sofa in the living room, so long as my legs were outstretched.

A story my father often told me is a good illustration of these habitual meetings with a cat. As a child, he lived with a cat known as "the Panther" because of the way she would lurk behind the front door and pounce on the women's skirts, causing them to cry out, which seemed to amuse her greatly. When my father went to bed, the Panther would go with him, stretch out on the bed, purr, and allow herself to be stroked. Then suddenly she would get up, press her muzzle against his cheek like a good-night kiss, and leave. One time when he tried to hold her back, he got a sharp swipe of the paw, which taught him that it was all about affection offered, not constraint.

I'm sure there are tens of thousands of you who could tell the tale of a rendezvous with your feline by heart. When that isn't the case, when the relationship is complicated, we prescribe a meeting therapy. The idea is to check on your cat's preferences and offer it the possibility of encountering its human companions at a particular time and place.

With this all-around treatment, Isis became a calm cat, and Aline and Raymond gained more cuddles and an improved relationship.

The Cat's Place in the Family

The case of Isis raises the question of the place that we accord to the cats in our lives.

Our common ground with cats resides in the possibility of mutual attachment: it enables relationships that give meaning and flavor to life. And no doubt we too have our own dual nature as predator and prey, buried deep but liable to make a reappearance. Not a very good predator in practice until we invented weapons to help us but, like cats, able to compensate for our physical weakness and low-grade natural defenses with a very advanced level of cognitive development.

What we cannot do, what we must not do, is ask our domestic cats to live and behave like little dogs. If we take the time to think like a cat—and that is the main purpose of this book—then the principles of a harmonious collaboration begin to become clear, and we all, cats included, have much to gain.

Putting ourselves in the place of cats involves, for example, not forcing them to live in company with other cats when they don't want to. Here again, there are always exceptions to the rule: cats who live in large colonies and who seem to thrive on it; cats who live alone and seem to suffer because of it. Nevertheless, I am much more in demand as a vet for cats who cannot stand living together than for cats who find being the only nonhuman animal in the house onerous.

On average, when the French own cats, they generally have more than one (1.68 to be precise). Since fractions of cats don't exist, that means that if you question five cat owners, they will have on average eight cats between them. Multi-cat households are quite common, and this communal existence can lead to behavioral issues.

"Charlie's Angels": Chérie and Kiss

Béatrice lived in a very smart Parisian apartment of more than 1,400 square feet. She contacted me about fisticuffs between two of the three cats in the household: Chérie and Kiss. Their fights didn't lead to injuries, even if the fur sometimes flew, but they were very noisy. And yet there was never any aggression between Charlie, the third cat of the household, and the other two cats.

Since Béatrice did not think it would be possible to bring all three cats into the practice (she described an epic visit to the vet with Kiss), she asked if it would be possible to do a video consultation. The protocol for vets in France is quite strict and is in the interests of the animals. No initial consultations by video: the physical examination is rightly held to be paramount. There is, however, one possibility: if a cat has been seen less than a month ago by the vet who is treating it, the latter can vouch for it and request the assistance of the veterinary specialist, who can conduct a teleconsultation legally. As in the case of Choupette, I could make a virtual visit to the apartment without frightening any of the cats, guided by Béatrice. She first introduced me to Charlie, a large ginger cat resting in sphinx pose in an armchair. Then we saw a ball of lighter-colored fur pass by and take refuge under another chair.

"Ah, that was Chérie! She's gone to hide under a chair, because Kiss is nearby."

A few seconds later, I saw a house cat turn up, walking slowly, head pointed toward the place where the other cat had disappeared.

Now I had seen all three protagonists.

Chérie was a small Ragdoll cat of five months. We have already met Tabatha in this book, who was of that same breed—the one who tilted at windmills. These cats have very soft fur and a coat resembling that of the Birman, with Siamese coloring (light body and dark face) and pretty white socks.

Like Tabatha, Chérie had been chosen for her breed's reputation for gentleness, even passivity, but let us reiterate: even though they are meant to be as manipulable as a rag doll, no cat should be transported or manhandled unceremoniously. The absence of an aggressive reaction doesn't signify well-being; in fact, inhibition is all too often a feline response that masks unease. Their mute suffering is not demonstrative enough, and the humans who live with them often fail to notice these silent symptoms. It is no doubt the main reason why we get relatively few such cats brought to us for consultation.

The Difficulty of Living Together

The role of the vet is crucial in bringing about change: they can explain that any reduction in activity can be a sign of behavioral issues and should not be ignored. Cats licking themselves to the point of losing their fur or bulimic cats whose obesity and failure to follow diets reveals a permanent anxious state are examples of pathological inhibition that require a subtle response from both owner and vet.

Luckily, this was not the case with Chérie, who bucked the trend for her breed and turned out to be a very active little cat. In fact, although she was quite placid with Béatrice, she was somewhat intrusive with the other two cats. She would allow herself to be carried by Béatrice, but would struggle after a few seconds and want to return to her activities, which consisted largely of hiding and leaping on the other cats.

While Charlie was quite accepting of the sometimes rough-and-tumble kitten games, this was not at all the case with fourteen-year-old Kiss, who tended to react badly to the inopportune "attacks" by the young female cat and defended herself by hissing and spitting. The aggressive reaction didn't deter Chérie, who simply returned to the fray. When Kiss spotted her, she would try to chase her from her sight and, if possible, from her territory. As they lived in an apartment, this was complicated, and Béatrice was starting to worry:

"The thing is, Doctor, it's already happened before! A few years ago, I wanted to get another cat, and as a precaution I asked to have a trial period to see if Kiss would accept her, but poor old Gwen didn't last a week! Kiss chased her, bit her, injured her, and I had to give her back."

"Yes, for some cats sharing their territory is a fraught business. But we can't generalize. Look at your Charlie—he seems to accept everyone. He is a very sociable cat. Kiss, on the other hand, has trouble defining her territory if another cat invades it and engages in marking. And if, on top of this, the young cat lacks self-control and does not respect the resident cat's demands to keep her distance, then there is very little chance of harmonious cohabitation."

How many times have I said that in my life, as I have tried to explain that the behavior of cats is different from that of a social species: as much as they are able to form very strong relationships with another individual, especially from another species, or with another cat, nothing is a given, and the relationship needs to fulfill certain conditions that are often not met.

Such failures of cohabitation are a source of disappointment to people who in good faith want to please their cats by providing them with company. I once heard a listener who called a radio program say that she had let her cat have a litter and had kept a kitten so that she would be less alone. The first four or five months went well but, after that, relations began to deteriorate, and the mother no longer tolerated her son, hissing at him, attacking him, refusing to play with him, and began to display signs of anxiety. It is easy to understand why her owner felt disillusioned and couldn't understand what seemed to her to be a dereliction of maternal love. While it is not known for sure, we are more or less certain that mothers recognize their kittens and behave with them in a particular way during the first weeks,[11] but after a few months the maternal relationship fades away and disappears. The son or daughter becomes just another adult cat who might be considered as much an intruder as any other cat. It seems incomprehensible to us, but is normal in the cat world. As was the case with Chérie and

Kiss, the young cat does not stop soliciting its mother, who rejects its demands. The confrontation between an individual who suffers from a lack of self-control and another with a tendency toward anxiety creates a situation of malaise for both, a malaise that family ties cannot appease.

Let's return to our lovely Parisian apartment. Kiss is a house cat. She arrived in the apartment after Charlie, who welcomed her with kindness. They shared their territory. I have already highlighted the importance of zones of isolation, the cat's secure territory, which the other living creatures should respect. Charlie had chosen an armchair, and Kiss never wanted to occupy that particular space. She chose instead the cat tree and the sofa, and Charlie didn't contest her choice. When Béatrice went to bed at night, she was often joined by Kiss, who would curl up next to her, satisfying her need for contact without being touched. As Béatrice had told me, Kiss had already refused to share her living space with another cat: the experiment had lasted only a few days but had failed miserably. Béatrice thought that maybe it was because she had made a mistake by trying to introduce an adult cat. Convincing herself that a kitten would benefit from diplomatic immunity, and having fallen in love with this cute and funny little Ragdoll, she attempted the experiment again.

"At first, I thought it had worked. I could see that Kiss didn't like her, I know she doesn't like other cats, but she carefully avoided her and spent a lot of time up high on the cat tree. Chérie couldn't join her there."

"How was Charlie? Did he play with the little one?"

"Charlie was an angel. Although I could see that Chérie pushed it too far, he was amazing. He played a little, did not threaten her, and even sometimes tried to hold her between his paws when she became too agitated. When that happened, I intervened and shut Chérie up in another room."

"How did the situation degenerate?"

"One day, Chérie jumped on Kiss as she came out of the bedroom. It was just overexuberant play, but Kiss reacted very badly. She hissed and started chasing the kitten and gave her a swipe with her paw. If I hadn't been there, I think she could have injured her."

"And how did Chérie take it?"

"I got the feeling she didn't know what was going on. Five minutes later, she was ready to do it again, and then she started following Kiss everywhere, wanting to sleep near her. The more Charlie indulged her, the less Kiss tolerated her."

"And things went from bad to worse?"

"Yes! I separated them once I realized that Kiss could injure her, and since then all hell has broken loose. Although there is enough space in the apartment for three cats, I have to make sure I close all the doors, but every now and again I make a mistake, and Kiss goes after Chérie."

Very Different Relations

This case is a classic one, and revealing in the way it evolved. Once again, we make an error when we think that an adult, especially a female, will be more tolerant of a baby than of an adult. Even if that is the case, essentially, with their own kittens, it is not generally true of other little ones. Tolerance toward infants affords important immunity to young ones. This is well known among social species, of which we are one, along with dogs and wolves, but does not exist among cats, as a nonsocial species. We have discovered that female cats are capable of adding a kitten to their litter, especially if they already have experience of motherhood.[12] In the wild, groups of females can form to share the care for kittens,[13] but one cannot assume that they would accept another individual under different circumstances.

It's fairly traumatizing for clients who fear for the life of their kitten when they witness the attacks unsociable adult cats are capable of. Unlike dogs, cats are not wired to accept the "other." The work we must do to understand and represent their world requires greater effort, but an empathetic approach also helps us to find solutions by respecting the way they function. And so I was able to explain to Béatrice that Kiss was not "mad" in any way, and even though the attacks showed that the relationship with Chérie was difficult, we were still within the bounds of the normal.

One has to assess all behaviors and, in a case like this, not just of one animal but three, without forgetting the interactions between each of the cats and the human protagonists. This semiological process often surprises clients, who think that we will only be dealing with the problematic behavior. We do address it at the start in order to get a sense of direction but then set it aside in order to look at all the other elements of an animal's behavior. The more complete the picture we form, the better our chances of identifying the pathological state of the animal, the relevant neurotransmitters, and the degree of the original behavioral disorganization to come up with a diagnosis, a prognosis, and a treatment.

Shared Territory, Complicated Cohabitation

In the case of "Charlie's Angels," the diagnosis didn't cause major problems. The suffering stemmed from the relationship (schezipathy) between two cats (intraspecies) and was related to the division of territory (biotopathy). Nowadays, we refer to this as an intraspecies *biotoschezipathy*. I spoke earlier about the anxiety of cohabitation, and if the theory of issues related to cohabitation was the correct one, then the two cats were not in a permanent anxious state. We saw the whole gamut of psychopathological states: from the normal, reactional one to phobic, anxious, or depressive states. This systemic diagnosis is not the end of the practitioner's work; they must also establish the diagnosis of each animal. While Charlie did not display any issues—being too easygoing is not abnormal—it wasn't obvious that this was the case for Kiss and Chérie.

The distinction between normal and pathological raises the question of limits. Having assessed her behaviors, I could confirm that Chérie needed to improve her self-control but we could not diagnose whether she was suffering from HSHA. It was the same for Kiss: her self-possession was fragile and she had doubtless suffered from lack of stimulation in her development, but nevertheless she was situated in the broad category of "still normal." We could establish this because, for example, the characteristics of her sleeping indicated neither anxiety nor depression. They all slept and dreamed, but Kiss had to "repel all boarders" on the bed, according to Béatrice's expression. The old cat had to chase Chérie every evening. They all still played. The three cats ate well and regularly. There was no urinary marking or excessive scratching. All three cats left their facial marking on inanimate objects and on Béatrice.

Loving Doesn't Always Mean Touching

Kiss could not stand to be touched for very long. If Béatrice tried to carry her, she was liable to struggle and scratch. Even when it was Kiss herself who sought the contact, after being stroked once or twice she might hiss and walk away or raise a threatening paw. By becoming habituated to contact through gentle stroking even while still inside the mother's belly, a cat is able to tolerate and appreciate our caresses. All kittens who have developed through this early contact (the sense of touch is in place at least two weeks before the kitten is born) have been found to be highly tolerant of forms of touch that we might assume would be unpleasant or almost painful to them. When a cat bites after being stroked, this always leads to a great misunderstanding on the part of humans, who are convinced that their cat must be duplicitous or fickle: it scratches or bites even though it asked for contact. We have to explain again and again that, for cats, being attached does not mean that they like to be touched. If they come and lie down next to you, that is already a major sign that they find you calming and that you provide them with a sense of security. Kiss displayed this intolerance of contact that is an indication of an absence of contact at an early stage of her development but not proof of an anxious state.

It is, of course, the encounter between a cat of an anxious predisposition with one that lacks self-control that favors the emergence of conflict, but when the semiology tells us that no one is ill, then we know that the prognosis is good.

So we put together a therapy and, as is usually the case with cats, this was environmentally based. We needed to reestablish the harmony of the biotope for each cat by locating and instilling respect for the different zones described in chapter 2. The zone of isolation is especially important for a cat, particularly those with anxious tendencies, who are even less willing than most to share.

There are various measures with varying degrees of sophistication. If the cat is microchipped and the owners can afford it, we recommend the use of an electronic cat flap that opens only for their cat as it returns to its place of security; it very soon learns that it will no longer be disturbed there.

As with Lucifer, we used a stimulus disruptor—a water pistol or a compressed-air keyboard cleaner—to interrupt Kiss's attacks on Chérie without punishing her. The disruption is not a punishment. It gives the cat a chance to escape somewhere else, and it is possible as a follow-up to suggest redirecting its activity toward a toy, even if that is not always easy.

Restructuring the environment, interrupting and redirecting aggressive behaviors, no more punishments—this is how most of our feline therapies are constructed.

As we have seen, Chérie and Kiss were not suffering from definite pathological states but they each had tendencies: hyperactivity for Chérie, anxiety for Kiss. In our treatment, then, we would use different nutraceuticals for each of them. For Chérie, a milk protein, alpha-lactalbumin, which is rich in tryptophan. It is a precursor of serotonin, a cerebral neurotransmitter that acts on control mechanisms. For Kiss, another milk-based protein, alpha-casozepine, a structural analog of GABA, a major neurotransmitter in the control of anxious states. If it hadn't already been tried out, we would have added a pheromone diffuser, but as Béatrice had already experimented for several weeks without success, we didn't insist on it.

After six weeks, things had improved significantly, and so quickly that Béatrice did not need to buy an electronic cat flap. Having grasped the underlying principle, she simply made her bedroom a sanctuary to which only Kiss had access. The way this cat sleeps there now, on her back and relaxed, confirms that she feels totally secure.

There were a few follow-up courses of treatment, and to consolidate the improvements we added for both animals one drop of hemp oil in the mouth, on the gingivolabial fold, morning and evening. This recently authorized supplement is a relaxant and in some cases boosts self-control mechanisms.

It's been good news ever since then, and the aggressive behavior has stopped. Béatrice has suggested that, although the situation has improved and there is no more danger, she is not sure whether Kiss—an old cat whom she wants to protect above all—will be happy as long as there is an intruder in the house. So she is considering whether or not to keep Chérie, but now that the cats are functioning together, she has time to reflect on this at her leisure.

*　　　*　　　*

Getting cats to live with others is never a foregone conclusion. They are capable of forming very intense bonds, but also of suffering with the same intensity from imposed relationships. Once one understands this, we can explain to our clients that when it comes to relationships involving cats everything is possible but nothing is obligatory. If it feels obligatory, the risk of it becoming a negative experience for the cat increases.

Isis was testament to the fact that living together is not always easy when, at every moment, there is the risk of misinterpretation. "Charlie's Angels" demonstrated that, even within a species, the superposition of living spaces, imposed cohabitation, can lead to tension. Fortunately, most of the time we can understand and resolve conflicts through a combination of empathy for both humans and felines, necessary tweaks to the environment, appropriate therapies, and a specially adapted therapeutic care package.

4

One Flew Over the Cat's Nest

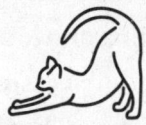

All cats are mortal. Socrates is mortal. Therefore, Socrates is a cat.

—*Eugène Ionesco*

Can cats be "mad"? We have already explored several areas of cat behavioral pathology: their relationships, their living space, even their predatory nature expose them to many problems that require veterinary intervention to reestablish their emotional balance. This all falls within the framework of what used to be called neuroses before the terminology evolved a few years ago. This term incorporated all the pathological states connected to the difficulty of living and adapting according to the individual personality of each animal and its environment. We are talking here about those phobic, anxious, and depressive states that make up the vast majority of our consultations, especially if one includes the lack of self-control that one finds in HSHA or aschezia. All these cats are still rooted in reality, even if the world they perceive is very different from ours, which requires an effort of imagination and lateral thinking on our part.

We are talking about whether it is possible for domestic cats to suffer from psychosis. This is a blanket term for all those states in which a disconnection from reality can be demonstrated, and it is in such cases that we can talk about a "mad cat." The term "madness" has become controversial in human mental health, and I have put it in quotation marks to express a certain caution, even though everyone knows what it means.

Feline Psychopathology

In his book *Folies animales* (*Animal Madness*), the emeritus professor of ethology Michel Kreutzer touches on an idea psychiatric vets have been proposing since the founding of Zoopsy (the Association of Veterinary Zoopsychiatry) in 1999.[1] He asserts that once you concede that other animals— at least some of them—have a psychological dimension, then there is no denying the existence of psychopathology in animals. He is here drawing on Henri Ey, who was the first to define the term *zoopsychiatry*.[2] Ey warned against simply transposing ideas about behavior from one species to another, and advocated that each species must therefore require its own particular psychiatry. It's an interesting approach, but it strikes me as only half true. Zoopsychiatry is the natural offspring of ethology and of the science of the behavior of all species in all their richness and diversity as well as of the psychopathological processes that are common to all of them and that vary in importance according to the ethogram (the sum of known behaviors pertaining to a species). For example, in prey species heightened sensitivity is a useful and natural phenomenon, but it can become a problem when it loses its adaptive quality and causes the animal to feel disproportionately fearful.

The combination of the two, normal behavioral repertoire and pathological processes, creates a different form of zoo-psychiatry for each species, with a number of common features that offer the practitioner ways to represent mental illnesses in any given species. For example, the semantic exercise carried out a few years ago around the terms for cat disorders, which I have touched on in previous chapters (biotopathy, schezipathy, and so on), has been very handy when looking at other species such as horses or rabbits. Although this is a work in progress, early research done by our students for their dissertations has indicated a way to harmonize veterinary psychiatric terminology in all the species we take care of. We can thus begin to trace a line between problems relating to everyday challenges and ones relating to a loss of contact with reality.

Still, this doesn't answer the question: Can cats be mad? It is striking to what extent philosophers, biologists, and ethologists find this notion of madness unacceptable, as if it had to be the preserve of humans, as if they alone might suffer from mental illness. Despite all its negative connotations, the term cannot be applied to the animal kingdom, it seems.

Psychiatric vets maintain the opposite: we believe that each animal species, in its representation of the world, and each member of that species, in its representation of itself in the world, can encounter pathological states in which their connection with reality is altered or lost. We call these "states of derealization," which can occur in various mental illnesses, and that is something we can term madness. For us, this is a label for a severe disorder involving a loss of contact with reality.

The use within veterinary psychiatry of the term "madness" does not refer to what some refer to as animal madness, which has nothing to do with that loss of contact with reality on the part of an individual belonging to a given species and living in a particular environment. The infanticides perpetrated by dolphins, monkeys, and lions are unrelated to madness even if they shock us, because we have forgotten that it was a fairly common practice among kings and in almost every civilization to kill the children of rivals who might have a claim on the throne. Infanticide in these species also poses the question of the recognition of their own young and the strategy used by a female to sow trouble in the mind of her male mate and protect her offspring. None of these sometimes subtle, sometimes violent, but always comprehensible adaptations involve loss of contact with reality; on the contrary, they once again break down the barrier that some people want to maintain at any cost between humans and other animals by showing that they too can have strategies for building dynasties. Today, there is even a theory that the mothers themselves take part in these infanticides, which shows how complex animal brains are. This behavior, which seems so strange and incomprehensible to us, is not restricted to the human species, even if, as far as I know, no lion, dolphin, or chimpanzee mother has had her son's eyes gouged out and left him to die of his wounds like Irene, mother of Constantine VI, to gain the throne of Byzantium.

There is a distinction between behavior that may strike us as unreasonable but which has its own logic, and madness, which can cause suffering and a detachment from the shared reality of the species.

Animal Testimonies

Once again, I will summon witnesses: cats who will show us how their very altered perception of reality can lead to major psychological issues. These cats are mad, and it is my mission—sometimes a desperate one—to take care of them. Of course, in human beings the dimension of speech adds to the feeling of strangeness, but if we project ourselves into the world of our domestic felines, we can see that they also suffer because of their inability to understand what is going on inside and around them and to communicate it.

As a practitioner I think I am allowed to say that cats can be "mad," like dogs, like parrots, but also like certain wild animals. In *Au risque d'aimer* (The Danger of Loving), my book on attachment and its possible excesses, I describe the moving story of Kamuniak, the lioness in Kenya who made headlines by protecting a baby oryx at Christmas 2001. Her behavior was admired at first (locals called her "Blessed"), but it began to be disturbing when she started stealing other baby oryxes and her passion seemed to turn into madness.[3]

In the book, I also give the example of Tilikum, the male orca responsible for three of the four fatal accidents recorded over a period of forty years in aquatic parks. There was a famous short film that featured him as a symbol of the mistreatment of these creatures in large aquatic parks.[4] It is not my intention here to defend this type of place, far from it, but I wish to apply a bit of scientific reasoning: if living conditions alone were enough to explain this, then there would have been many more Tilikums and many more accidents.

This killer whale seemed to have very high cognitive abilities, something spotted by his warden, Dawn Brancheau, an expert whale trainer, who would be his final victim. She recognized Tilikum's exceptional abilities, which were well above those of the average orca in her experience. But at times he could literally become "mad," with sudden changes of mood and unconstrained dangerous behavior. When the accident happened, she had warned fellow staff that he was having a bad day. On closer inspection, one can see evidence of the type of bipolar disorder that we discussed earlier in relation to Nougatine. In her case it was severe but not extreme and she remained connected to reality; it seems that Tilikum had suffered crises on at least three previous occasions that made him lose his bearings and led him to kill. I'm not denying that his environment could have aggravated matters: it seems to me that, as in my day-to-day practice, psychiatric pathology emerges out of both an individual vulnerability and an unfavorable environment, in varying proportions. Some disorders always show up, whatever the conditions; others, conversely, are very sensitive to the quality of the context—but there is always cross-participation.

Nougatine's bipolar dysthymia was a limit case of derealization—that is, an extreme disconnection from reality. In less serious cases, there is just an excessive reaction or conversely a loss of reactivity but the cat remains in connection with reality. This can even be normal, as is the case for us humans. Some involve a fairly constant mood, but many involve spontaneous variations of mood of short duration. When it becomes a little more pronounced, the term *cyclothymia* is used to designate this state where the joyful phases, sometimes bordering on hyperactivity, alternate with darker moments, imbued with unwarranted sadness or anhedonia (the inability to feel positive emotions).

When hyperactivity and hypoactivity both cross the threshold of normality, we vets talk about bipolar dysthymia, and this can be compared to human bipolar disorder. The most marked active episodes (with violent agitation and occasionally lethal attacks) sometimes lead us to label these extreme cases as severe psychiatric illnesses accompanied by states of derealization.

Tilikum is testimony to this, and his example makes the case not just for necessary changes in the conditions of captivity (at least until there are no longer orcas held in captivity) but also for treating with respect this individual who combined genius and madness.

Lisbeth: A Panther on a Prescription

Annie lived with Lisbeth, a pretty calico cat, before she met her partner Luc. When Luc moved in with Annie, it took Lisbeth a few months to accept him. The swipes of the paw, scratches, and unfriendly growls lasted nearly a year, eventually becoming less frequent and then giving way to a harmonious cohabitation. Luc and Lisbeth even enjoyed some caresses while watching the news on TV in the living room.

One day, Lisbeth had a sore mouth. Annie took her to the vet, who, as is often the case, used steroids to treat the inflammation. Normally, these work quickly and effectively. But here, no sooner had the soreness diminished than Lisbeth's mood suddenly deteriorated, and she became quite menacing. One evening, after Luc had been watching TV until late, he followed Annie to bed; Lisbeth made it known she didn't think it was a good idea by blocking the door and spitting and hissing. Thanks to their years living together and perhaps not wanting to show weakness, Luc went into the bedroom. Lisbeth hurled herself at him and scratched and bit him so badly he had to seek urgent medical care. It is worth pointing out that more people go to the hospital after being attacked by a cat than by a dog, even if they require less treatment. Some colleagues of mine who work as voluntary firefighters alongside their professional duties have described emergency calls where frightened owners have been trapped in bathrooms or out on balconies by their "mad" cats who are trying to attack them and who represent a genuine danger.

Controlled Moods

Steroids have anti-inflammatory properties but also act on mood and actively inhibit the function of the hypothalamic-pituitary-adrenal axis by negative feedback. The link between this axis, the administration of steroids, and the unleashing of psychoses is well known and has been the subject of numerous publications in human medicine.[5] In veterinary psychiatry, which sometimes has difficulty in holding its own and still lacks institutional university support to pursue this type of study, we are not there yet, but, though we must be cautious about simply transposing data on human cases to animal ones, there is no reason not to suspect that the same type of mechanism is at work in sudden and violent jolts of mood within animals.

In our day-to-day clinical life, cases such as Lisbeth's are not common but they occur often enough to give us pause for reflection. The treatments that act more or less directly upon the equilibrium of the hypothalamic-pituitary-adrenal axis (such as the steroids mentioned above, including certain progestogens—such as megestrol acetate) and some antiemetics (metoclopramide) can induce—on rare occasions but spectacularly—the equivalent of what might be termed a "psychotic episode" with a loss of contact with reality and a sudden and unpredictable increase in dangerousness.

We have indirect evidence of the involvement of the hypothalamic-pituitary-adrenal axis during these episodes when using a dopaminergic product that we know acts at the level of the hypothalamus and can restore a degree of mental balance. It is necessary to administer the product to a cat that is out of control and potentially very dangerous. Amazingly, there is often one person, the main figure of attachment, who is spared during these crises. This was the case with Lisbeth. Annie remained safe. She couldn't do everything, of course, but she was able to dispense the medicine without being instantly torn to shreds. Such cases are very impressive: I always admire the courage of owners who choose to care for their cats in such conditions. Earlier, we talked about Nougatine and Catherine's family, where the attacks were not so serious, but the family nonetheless required perseverance and boldness. Here the prognosis is much better, the crisis is iatrogenic: that is to say that the symptoms are related to the administration of medication (the steroid meant to address Lisbeth's sore mouth). When its effect has passed, we are hopeful that the situation will return to normal. In addition, by administering the right treatment, we will shorten the episode by a month or just over a fortnight at the most. This was the case for Lisbeth: she was confined to the kitchen, and Annie was able to give her the tablet, which was a real feat. In the first fortnight, whenever Luc went past the glazed door, Lisbeth would hiss and throw herself with claws exposed at his silhouette.

Side Effects to Consider

You need to be very attached and determined to keep your cat in order to accept such a dangerous situation: sometimes we suggest hospitalizing the cat for a few days or weeks, to allow some time for its mood to become normal again. Nowadays, most vets know what can happen when administering certain medications, but this very undesirable side effect is sufficiently rare that sometimes we can forget to report it to the cat's owners. Knowing this does not enable us to prevent the episode (we don't measure the size of the pituitary gland or the impact of steroids on the hippocampus), but it does enable us to react quickly and say: "It's unusual but it can happen. Keep yourself safe. If you can, put your cat into its carrier and bring it in to the clinic: we will take care of it!"

It's the only way to protect the owners and especially the cat, for whom otherwise the only option is euthanasia, given the extent to which such an episode can undermine the confidence of those who live with it.

Lisbeth was lucky enough to live with Annie, who couldn't contemplate being separated from her, especially when she learned that her cat's transformation into a voracious panther in relation to Luc was temporary. She hung in there, sought treatment for Lisbeth, and managed to protect both her partner and her cat. Three weeks later, harmony was restored. Lisbeth and Luc had reinstated their cuddles in front of the TV, even if Luc understandably continued to be nervous. For her part, Lisbeth seemed to forget that, for a few days, and under the strange effects of her medication, she became the prescription panther.

The vet merely had to note on her patient form that she was prone to mood swings, dysrhythmic episodes, following the use of certain products that had to be proscribed for her.

Madness can be induced by medication, which shows us that mental and physical health are not separate categories but there is a single general balance in which everything is connected. Some may say that this provoked madness is not a real "autonomous" illness, but they are overlooking a whole host of other illnesses that are set off by certain treatments. No one would tell a patient that an infection they contracted in the hospital is not a real disease when its sometimes fatal severity and prognosis are today a matter of concern for the entire medical profession. However, you can be sure that, just as Kamuniak or Tilikum attest to the existence of madness in the wild, there will also be evidence of spontaneous "madness" among our domestic cats.

Even now, we can note to what extent the nonsocial structure of the feline species modifies behavioral issues. Familiarization is gained from experience, it is not a natural predisposition of the feline species, and it is often the first thing to be affected, while attachment, which is different and much deeper by nature, can sometimes be respected even in a loss of contact with reality. But beware: in other cases, even the cat's special person can also be in danger, so the bond cannot always be relied upon for protection. It can in one respect, however: it is the reason that the human who lives with the cat asks us to try all we can to control these states. Without attachment, the issue would be fatal for the animal much more frequently.

Consulting the Veterinary Psychiatrist

When Nathalie called to make some inquiries, I sensed that she hadn't made up her mind whether to come and see me. She described to me a cat with changeable behavior and chronic skin disorders marked, among other things, by alopecia (fur loss, which had made the skin visible) on its back. A number of veterinary dermatologists had looked into it, but they too had ended up tearing their hair out (figuratively speaking) and giving up because the case was so complex. The last one she consulted, who often referred clients to me, had advised her that psychological balance might be a possible factor.

Today, there are veterinary hospitals with teams of different specialists capable of carrying out every kind of medical and surgical procedure, and veterinary psychiatrists are gradually becoming included. This enables fruitful exchanges, when they can be set up, and we are all aiming to achieve a better quality of medical care by combining these highly specialized skills with treating the individual as a whole and in relation to their environment. This is the "one health" concept of medicine, which asks us not to lose sight of the link among all the organs inside the body and the link between the body and the other living beings around it and with its environment as a whole. Fortunately, we didn't have to wait for these advances for many colleagues to start thinking along these lines and asking us to become involved when a physical condition proved resistant to treatment.

There I was, on the phone with Nathalie: she wasn't hostile, but she was skeptical. I have to admit that, after thirty years of repeating the same explanations, I sometimes forget that my listener is hearing them for the first time. "You're going to do what? How are you going to do that? You're sure you're able to do something? She's not in a crisis now, so you won't see anything." It is difficult not to interpret such skepticism as a vote of no confidence when, in the vast majority of cases, it simply reflects a genuine concern. I have to repeat patiently that, as in all medical disciplines, thanks to our information gathering, thanks to our behavioral semiology, we are able to make a diagnosis.

Cardiologists don't need to run alongside their patients; nor do dermatologists, whether for humans or animals, need to be covered in papules or pustules to understand what their patient is suffering from.

Cause and Request

Medical procedure is at the heart of our practice as psychiatric vets, and since our consultations are still something of a mystery to many, let us recap how they work.

First, we hear the cause of the problem often expressed as a complaint by the humans who accompany the cat: "He is dirty . . . he is aggressive . . ." That points us in the right direction but never provides an immediate answer. Whatever the evidence seems to be saying, we always need confirmation.

Cause is one element, request is another. It's probably what makes the most difference between veterinary psychiatry and other disciplines, even if there are some similarities with those disciplines that often have to grapple with chronic diseases, with significant investment (both in time and money) and with an uncertain prognosis (dermatology, oncology, dietetics, etc.).

The same cause can hide behind very different requests. Let us take the example of a dirty cat that regularly soils parts of the house and deposits smelly traces of urine. The most obvious request is "Make it stop!" But that is not always the case. Sometimes it has been going on for so long that the owners are resigned and just want to reassure themselves that it is not a sign that their cat is in a bad way. (Well, in fact, yes, it is.) Or else, and it is more bothersome and crucial to identify it quickly, behind the cause given there is sometimes a desire to be rid of an animal that has become unwanted, too distant from the fantasy its human companions had in their head or too much of a disruption to social and family life.

Often, the exact way they frame their request gives an insight into how far the owners are prepared to go: Do they have enough energy to put new solutions in place? Are they sad, exhausted, desperate, exasperated? Or full of hope and ready to try again? It can be difficult to gauge the right amount of time to devote to the request: not enough, and the client does not feel properly heard and doesn't understand the course of treatment; too much, and there is a risk of their drowning in detail given prematurely.

A Full Picture

When we have allocated the right amount of time to this part of the consultation, semiological research during the next stage is particularly important. The role of the vet here is to translate: they must transform the signs, every detail provided by the owner, however naive or trivial, into symptoms recognizable by all practitioners, connected if possible to the involvement of a particular neurotransmitter, which puts us on the trail of the correct medication, the exact diagnosis, or the adapted therapy. Our consultations are long, but they aren't just a chat: the transformation of these signs into symptoms by the alchemy of science allows the practitioner to build up a picture of the condition. Our position is a constructivist one, in line with the ideas of the Austrian-American psychologist and philosopher Paul Watzlawick: "Constructivist psychotherapy is not the illusory belief that it will make the client see the world as it really is. On the contrary, constructivism is fully aware that this new vision of the world is, and cannot fail to be, another construction, another fiction, but a useful vision, a less painful one."[6]

The psychiatric vet constructs on the basis of the assembled symptoms a representation of the reality they will refer to when moving forward with the client and with the cat. It is not surprising that two practitioners can come up with two different yet equally effective constructions, even though the range of possibilities is not infinite.

The vet explores all the behaviors of the animal, not just the problem behavior. The other parts of the behavioral repertoire allow us to discern more clearly the animal's functioning at the neurotransmitter level, a fundamental understanding that makes for better prescribing. We review all the "centripetal" behaviors, those regarding the relationship of the animal to its own body—food, drink, sleep, disposal, cleaning—and then the "centrifugal" ones: relationships with others, play with other individuals, agonistic behaviors (fight and flight), and especially exploratory behavior. Finally, we examine mixed behaviors, those that concern both the animal's body and its relationship with the world and with others, which the cat has in abundance: marking, attachments, sexual and maternal behavior if the animal has not been spayed or neutered.

Once all the behaviors have been assessed, it is important to assess the history of the cat's development, including any medical episodes that may have occurred and that can be potential triggers for behavioral issues, and, whenever we can, we always perform a physical examination, which may not seem necessary but can be a source of useful information.

This is why a feline psychiatric consultation (and it's the same if not more intensive for dogs) can't be over and done with in ten minutes. Understanding the best form of intervention is achieved by gaining an intimate knowledge of the life of Moustache, Flora, or Belzébuth, of the cat who is there in front of us, and not through general and superficial information. Remember all the possible combinations of the dual prey–predator nature of the cat and you will understand why the procedure has to be highly individualized even if it follows general principles.

Behavioral Therapy

Having reached a diagnosis, the psychiatric vet will then share it with their client and get them to agree with what is proposed. If there is no shared vision, the chances of success are minimal. We must always take the time to explain, using metaphors and images to help, where necessary, for example to convince owners of the need for medication for their cat, which is something that may take them a while to digest.

Once we have a consensus on the nature of the problem and how to treat it, the vet can prescribe, write down the details of the therapy (how many pills or drops, how many times a day, how to dispense them), and also, most importantly, provide an explanation of the behavioral therapy. With cats, as we have seen, that almost always begins with an end to physical punishment—and don't raise your eyebrows if you have never dreamed of giving your cat a slap. If you could be a fly on the wall during my consultations, you would be amazed to hear how many people have punished or smacked their cat, rubbed the cat's nose in its feces, yelled, and so on. I often give the example of a lady of a certain age, a professional woman, who admitted that she hit her cat with a telephone directory: "I read in a detective novel that it doesn't injure, it doesn't leave a mark, but it does make a strong impression." It certainly made an impression on me . . . and no doubt the cat.

When owners confide in us like this, it is because they understand that we aren't there to judge them but to help them (which doesn't mean that we agree with them about everything, and certainly not about telephone directories). They give us a lot of precious and precise information that we can put to good use in the treatment, and we are very often thankful to them for giving us all these details, which proves that they trust us.

So the diagnosis is established, the treatment prescribed. But the most important part for the person who lives with the animal is the prognosis. Is the illness treatable? How long will it take? How much will it cost? What is the likelihood of success? All legitimate questions that we are able to answer as our treatment progresses.

Essential Follow-Up

Finally, we need to sort out the follow-up. We are not magicians and, depending on the diagnosis, we have to accompany the owners in their work of behavioral therapy for as long as it takes. We've already touched on this in the case of Choupette, but nowadays teleconsultation has added an extra dimension to our practice, and especially when it comes to the follow-up. Some people talk about telemedicine as a poor substitute for the real thing, but in my experience it offers a different and complementary form of medicine.

Of course, it is impossible to do an accurate physical examination at a distance, even if it is only a matter of time and advances in technology before that becomes a possibility. I have already managed with some clients who were up for it to conduct tests on postural reflexes with their cat at home, which has allowed me to rule out certain neurological conditions. And besides, being able to observe a cat in its normal environment, without the presence of the vet being a major intrusion, and without obliging it to travel to a strange place where it will feel ill at ease, is a considerable plus. The follow-up allows us to assess how the condition is developing, firstly from a global point of view, then by checking all the elements that were dysfunctional in the first consultation, not forgetting to see whether anything else has gone awry. This enables us to tweak the therapy. Observing the way that the home is organized allows us to identify elements that may not have been suspected at the time of the initial consultation and to finesse measures for changing the environment. A description of any noticeable or unusual side effects tells us how to adapt the therapy by changing the dose or rate of administration, or more often by not changing anything but simply explaining and reassuring.

To cure a behavioral issue or to alter a pathological state often requires several months, or at the very least several weeks, and the first consultation, no matter how good it was, will never be enough. It is the follow-up that enables a real cure. It is always a great moment when one can discharge a patient, with the objectives all achieved. This brings us back to differentiating between cause and request. One classic trap is that a shift occurs in the course of a follow-up: sometimes the original complaint is resolved, but, happy to see that change is possible, the owners might express other wishes. Then, it is crucial to record that the first goal has been achieved, that the initial request was satisfied, before deciding whether it is necessary to continue with a new objective.

These are things I should explain on every occasion, but I don't always have the time to say. Being able to do so in these pages will, I hope, serve to create a better understanding of the way psychiatric vets work, assuage uncertainties, and instill confidence in this new medical practice that tackles behavioral suffering in animals.

Melly Makes You Want to Pull Your Own Hair Out

Let's return to my phone call with Nathalie; she was uncertain whether to proceed with a consultation. After a few minutes' chat, she understood that I was ready to listen, and we arranged a meeting.

The first thing that Nathalie said to me was: "Every time I've told my story to a vet, I've got the impression they thought I was crazy." I reassured her: "I hear that a lot, and it's understandable: animal psychiatry is not taught in veterinary college, and most vets are not qualified in this discipline. They are surprised to hear about symptoms they've never learned about and that don't mean anything to them. Tell me everything, but first of all introduce me to the young lady."

Nathalie placed a cat carrier on the table. When I approached, I saw that it contained a magnificent female Abyssinian cat. The origins of the breed are shrouded in mystery: Did it come from Ethiopia, as implied by the name, as well as by the legend of the first Abyssinian cat, Zula, who is said to have been brought back from Addis Ababa? Did the breed come from Asia? Or was it just the fruit of selection of cats with large ears and an oriental appearance?[7]

Even though I make the point again and again that belonging to a breed is not a predictor of behavior, I remain open to everything genetics can offer us, and, while breed is not a good indicator, it would be ridiculous to deny that some lineages (some families) share similar behavioral traits and even identical behavioral issues, which indicate either a genetic root or a common cause in development.

A Family Resemblance

Melly belonged to that breed of Abyssinians in which many lineages seem to suffer psychiatric problems marked by states of derealization. I wasn't too surprised at what Nathalie told me.

"In effect, I don't have one cat, I have two: adorable Melly, who is loved by everybody, and the little devil who scares us and sometimes hurts people."

I approached the door of the cat carrier; I talked to Melly in soothing tones and I observed her initial reactions. She came up to sniff me through the grille of the door and appeared to be calm. I opened the door and offered my immobile hand, at which the cat showed no signs of being frightened and didn't recoil, but when the door was opened wide, she left the carrier and stretched out on the table.

I touched her, and she rubbed herself against me, looking at me with an inquisitive expression, her tail up straight with only its tip slightly curled, a perfect question mark. It's a cat way of saying: "So what's this all about, then?"

"You see, I told you, you won't see a thing," Nathalie exclaimed, and I understood her frustration.

"Don't worry, I won't doubt what you tell me, and I can see on her back lighter areas where the fur has not grown back as it should."

"That's nothing, When I took her to the dermatologist, she had nothing but a line of hairs on her back."

"I believe you. I can see the area that must have been hairless, and I assume that Melly caused that with her licking."

"Absolutely! They had all sorts of theories: fleas! Imagine fleas in my house. . . ."

"It's far from the most likely cause of this type of lesion, and even cats in apartments can pick up fleas. . . ."

"It wasn't that. Nor was it a food allergy or any of the other things they tested for. And what baffled your colleagues the most were the flare-ups that weren't related to seasons. . . ."

"Okay! We'll now explore all her behaviors, and, for each of them, I want you to give me the two versions: when Melly is doing well and when she turns into a devil. . . ."

And so we began the semiological survey, where I reminded her we would review everything that made up the exact behavioral repertoire of this cat, or rather these two cats in the case of Melly and the two versions of her.

It was no surprise to find out that all the cat's major functions were affected by her problems. Food, first and foremost! Although Melly had a normal appetite most of the time, during her crises she alternately ate with a voracious appetite or else more or less stopped eating and seemed irritated. She would manage to crunch a little cat kibble, then run off as if she had just had an electric shock or just spotted a potential threat.

Although her drinking was little affected, her disposal behavior changed. Nathalie described to me a delicate and punctilious cat who carefully buried her waste in her periods of normality. In moments of crisis, although she herself remained more or less clean, she neglected to cover her excrement and would jump out of her litter box so quickly she would spill stools outside the box.

"Nothing was different in the apartment, but I always got the feeling she had the devil on her heels. An even more distressing feeling for Melly, as the 'devil' was inside her—she couldn't escape it no matter how hard she tried."

When we use the clients' own images it helps them to better grasp the representation of the illness, and hearing their own words makes it easier for them to take it on board. I didn't dwell on somesthetic behavior (cleaning, licking, and so on). We spoke about it at the beginning and we would return to it later, but I didn't want the whole of the semiological stage to be taken up by this one issue.

Journey to the End of the Night

I am interested in sleep—its quality, the places chosen by the cat, and the eventual acceptance of company.

"You'll need to ask Chouchou about that—he's the best one to talk to," Nathalie told me with a smile.

"Who is Chouchou?"

"Chouchou is my other cat . . . a six-year-old European, a neutered male. When everything is going well, in the normal periods, Melly sleeps between Chouchou's paws."

"Really? Are you sure?"

"Well . . . I do live with them all the time, you know."

"Yes, of course, forgive me."

My surprise was due to the fact that this behavior is somewhere between rare and nonexistent. In principle, only cats who are siblings or affiliated share the same zone of isolation. Not for the first time cats had shown they have precious little regard for theory. In the field of feline behavior, as we have seen, there are always many exceptions to the general rules.

Nathalie elaborated: "These days it's my usual indicator. When everything is okay, I often see them sleeping or resting together. Chouchou licks Melly, and she lets him, and then . . . suddenly, even though nothing seems to have happened, Chouchou leaps up to get away from Melly, and I know that a crisis is on the way."

I could then verify that the amount of sleep Melly was getting seemed reduced and the dream phases, which were barely perceptible in the normal periods, disappeared altogether.

Sleep is an important element in our semiology and is often overlooked. The location and quality of the zone of isolation are of interest, but, beyond that, the behavioral characteristics tell us a lot about the emotional state. Hyperactive cats sleep very little and either don't dream at all or dream very little; anxious cats wake up and move about; depressives wake with a start, progress to REM sleep, and feel anxious before going to sleep; while normal cats sleep a lot and are champions when it comes to dreaming.

The Science of Dreams

On our degree course in veterinary psychiatry we had the pleasure of welcoming Raymond Cespuglio, who worked with the famous neurobiologist Michel Jouvet on defining REM sleep. In experiments that would no longer be authorized today, it was shown that this phase of dreaming corresponded to brain activity comparable to that of the waking state but in which muscle tone was almost wholly abolished by a small part of the brain called the locus coeruleus. When they cut away this exact area, researchers were able to observe the behaviors that populate cat dreams. They were surprised to find that, even in the gentlest animals, the most common behavioral sequences were attacks, followed by licking and the characteristic lying in wait.[8] The team was surprised not to observe any sexual behavior in these feline dreams, though the article didn't say whether the animals were spayed or neutered or in the estrus phase—in heat—which would otherwise explain why this activity did not occupy their nights, the frequency of erotic dreams in humans being related to sexual activity, which is permanent, unlike in other animals.

"Champions, gold medalists in dreaming": it was Boris Cyrulnik who coined this phrase in relation to cats. He even quoted a figure of 200 minutes of REM sleep for cats each night, as opposed to 100 minutes for humans. You can check for yourself, as I have, that these figures are correct.[9] Dreams are important in the maturing of babies' and infants' brains but also for emotional balance and ability to learn in adults. To such an extent that, as opposed to the received idea that dreams protect sleep, nowadays neurobiologists think that sleep is there to allow us to dream.

But why is dreaming so important for our domestic feline species? My theory is that, again, it has to do with its double nature as predator and prey. In a cat's life, there is a division between these two modes of activity, both of them vital but very different in nature. If we take the activities described by Jouvet's team, we see that all the lurking and hunting behavior belongs to the predator mode, while everything to do with defensive aggression and attack has to do with the prey mode. This leaves the third activity, somesthetic—that is, centered on the cat's body. The grooming routine, which can at times seem frenetic, shows the importance of good self-maintenance and no doubt the emotional impact of certain dream situations, with the cat soothing itself in a natural way by focusing on itself.

Here is another element to add to the already complex file of cats' cerebral functions. They dream, they dream a lot, and a lack of dreaming is an important semiological clue. In cats, remember, the motor inhibition in the course of the dream phase is stronger than in dogs—this is no doubt connected to their nature as prey. I have seen sleeping dogs wagging their tails in their dreams, mimicking what they do when they come into contact with another dog. In cats, the signs are much more subtle. Luckily for us, cat owners are often close observers of their companions and they give detailed descriptions of twitching whiskers, moving toes, ears pricked as if the cat is listening, and, above all, eyeballs moving in an uncoordinated manner beneath closed eyelids. It is this last point that is the origin of the name by which this sleep phase is known in the literature: rapid eye movement (REM), as opposed to the rest of sleep, known as the non–rapid eye movement phase (NREM).

When It All Goes Wrong

To return to our complicated cat, Nathalie described Melly in her angelic version, sleeping between the paws of Chouchou, in a shared and accessible zone of isolation and displaying several observable phases of dreaming. Conversely, in devil mode, Melly slept a lot less, never entered into REM sleep, and seemed very nervous and irritable, a sign of the profound change in the animal's emotional and cognitive economy.

Her exploratory behavior was also very different during these episodes: she prowled around the apartment, started at the slightest noise, and would "spit" in a threatening manner, as cats do when they are frightened.

Nathalie also flagged that Melly stopped playing when she was having a bad spell. Normally she would happily chase after rolled-up balls of silver foil or wait for her favorite human to play with her headphone wires in a welcoming ritual that could last for several minutes, but in her bad spells she did not respond to any solicitation, or sometimes even reacted in an aggressive way. She would growl at anyone and everyone, lash out with her paws, arch her back in a menacing way, with her fur standing up and her ears flattened on her head.

When Melly was in that state of mind, everything was a potential threat, and, like any vulnerable prey, she had to defend herself against everything, including her best friends.

We can readily imagine her suffering. In our work of empathy, picturing the change of environment that this dysfunctional brain provokes is a bit like being a child watching Snow White running through a forest pursued, in her fevered imagination, by the branches of the trees, which are trying to harm her. The sensation of terror that we experience must be very close to what Melly lived through. The three classic responses to intense fear are *fight*, *flight*, or *freeze* (already encountered earlier as the 3F rule). In Melly, the responses to her intense fears, which came from within but were no less real to her for that, were fight and flight. That didn't make her a "bad" cat; she was simply unwell.

Chouchou's reaction during these bad spells was characteristic; he didn't get angry with Melly. He recognized her, so he didn't mistake her for an unknown, aggressive cat.

Nevertheless, he sought safety and couldn't understand why his friend had suddenly changed behavior so radically. It's an element that I always integrate into my semiology, a way of taking account of how *other* animals react—a respect for their emotional intelligence. Chouchou seemed to be saying: "You know, sometimes Melly is really strange. . . ." And I totally agreed with him.

We came back to the problem behavior, the reason for these consultations: our patient's grooming behavior. Now that we had assessed the other symptoms, the main complaint of compulsive licking could be explained in a completely new way. Nathalie summed it up herself: "In fact, when Melly is in one of her bad phases, she does everything with abnormal intensity. Her fear, aggressivity, and vigilance are exacerbated: nothing is normal anymore."

An Illness I Recognize

When the semiological discussion goes well, it's not unusual that the client comes to the same conclusion as we do. All we need to do is to establish the diagnosis. These days, it is not always easy to distinguish between the two severe psychiatric disorders found in our domestic carnivores (and which exist *mutatis mutandis* in humans): bipolar dysthymia and dissociative syndrome. The former, which we have discussed in relation to Nougatine, leaves the animal connected to reality even if its reactions are disproportionate, but the latter plunges them into another world, one that we don't have access to and has few points of intersection with our reality. The sudden change that came over Melly, the fact that she seemed not to recognize anyone and others didn't recognize her, her estrangement from her normally familiar environment—all this inclines us toward a diagnosis of dissociative syndrome, an equivalent of human schizophrenia, found in dogs as well as cats.

Let's be clear: we are not saying that it is the same condition, that the psychotic episodes are identical. The world of a cat, its *Umwelt* (that is, its perception of the world and its representation of itself in this world), in other words everything that makes sense for a cat in its environment, is not the same as that of a human, so there is no reason to think that the episodes are the same. "Cats' dreams are full of mice," wrote the French mathematician René Thom, in an echo of Ludwig Wittgenstein's comment about lions. They are saying the same thing, only in different terms: the worlds of different species are not comparable, to which we would add that we need to factor in the uniqueness of each individual. Will technology one day allow us to make images of these losses of contact with reality? What huge colorful mouse or monstrous dog suddenly invades Melly's world and terrorizes her beyond anything we can imagine? What unbearable physical sensation causes her to lick herself to the point that she pulls out her fur, like that young woman who recounted how she tore out her hair during delirious episodes?[10]

Although human schizophrenia and feline dissociative syndrome are not interchangeable, they resemble each other, they are part of the same family of conditions that have their roots in an unregulated cerebral physiology. Genetic vulnerability, the influence of very early development or of food on the balance of gut microbiota, everything that interests doctors the most in the early detection of schizophrenia, and in its prevention, could one day soon form part of the diagnostic repertoire of the veterinary psychiatrist.

This requires a recognition of such feline disorders and the conviction that our pets, in their world, can also be mad.

Did You Say "Madness"?

If I happen to mention this notion at a workshop attended by a dozen or so vets, I am very often met with an initial marked skepticism or, at best, polite indifference. Then, when I describe the symptoms, it rings a bell; they remember clinical cases of their own, and are often convinced in the end. Indeed, in many cases they go on to refer animals to me with a note: "Dear colleague, I'm referring Romeo to you, as I believe he is presenting the two severe psychiatric conditions that I heard you describe." It's true that it is only possible to recognize something that you already know.

I'm in no doubt that in the years to come the treatment of these illnesses will improve. There is just one key element missing: veterinary colleges must open their doors to proper psychiatric training and not limit themselves, as they do now, to the teaching of ethology. It's as if the faculty of human medicine didn't speak about mental pathology but restricted itself to sociology—an interesting science, of course, but not of primary concern to doctors.

We are the doctors of nonhuman animals, and our oath, like the Hippocratic oath, enjoins us to relieve our patients' pain. We weren't at fault for failing to take mental suffering into account when the state of our knowledge did not allow us to contribute to the diagnosis and treatment of the psychiatric disorders of the animals delivered into our care, but we could potentially be in the future. Now that animal consciousness is at the heart of scientific research and well-being is a major preoccupation in our society, how can we ignore this whole level of animal suffering?

Learn More to Care Better

I presented the diagnosis to Nathalie, who was at once worried and relieved. Relieved because I validated her concerns. Worried because the diagnosis was alarming, and I couldn't give her much reassurance: I would prescribe a treatment, of course, but without being fully confident, because I couldn't see the bigger picture and didn't have all the tools at hand. Nevertheless, I knew that Melly's future was clearer, less because I knew how to cure her than because Nathalie, now that she knew her enemy, would be able to organize things better and was no longer struggling in the dark. At a time, in ancient Egypt, when physicians had just as few means at their disposal, they would say, "It's an illness I know and I can tell you the name," and this statement was their first therapeutic act.

The treatment was tough, and not helped by Melly's refusal to take medication. The crises were limited, and the balance between benefit and risk was not in favor of daily administration. After several weeks of trying, Nathalie gave up trying to treat Melly. I believe Chouchou would warn them when a crisis was brewing. At that moment, she would lock Melly in the calmest room possible for the protection of everyone, with no light, noise, or stimulation, which was in line with my behavioral therapy.

I received news of Melly from time to time. She died a few years later from kidney failure, like many cats regardless of whether they are suffering from a dissociative disorder. The case of Melly happened a long time ago, and, luckily, such cases are rare, though they are not exceptional. Often they are not picked up in the journey from dermatology to neurology, which sometimes ends in euthanasia. In the recent past I have seen a number of cats have their tails amputated after some very serious bouts of self-mutilation. Just the last third at the tip of the tail, but, if the animal is still in crisis, no collar or other means will resist its devastating "madness," and further mutilation will result in another amputation, as far back as the first caudal vertebrae. It is at this point, in the face of obvious suffering and with the therapy at a dead end, that the decision is often made to put the cat down for compassionate reasons. It is easy to understand those colleagues who, never having had any training in feline psychiatry, feel helpless in the face of this pain which is as much physical as psychological.

New Tools to Implement New Ideas

Nowadays, the question of suffering is still taxing. A century ago, the experience of pain was the subject of the same debate, and some people argued that animals had the same pathways, the same molecules signaling pain, but which they felt should be designated by a different word in order to distinguish humans from other animals. This nonsense has now been dispensed with, and now best practice in human medicine includes knowing how to manage pain on a day-to-day basis, from expedient measures to supporting old age through all types of painful conditions.

"But suffering is the same for all, isn't it?" I would ask as a newly qualified vet.

"Don't get carried away, young man! To suffer you must be conscious of your condition, be aware that it could be different, that there could, in a manner of speaking, be another life."

I confess I usually laugh at this, but it can sometimes be demoralizing. Thirty years later I keep encountering the same invisible barrier that shifts slightly from era to era but that tries to maintain a watertight seal between human beings and other animals.

Everyone these days talks about well-being, but few are willing to grant cats the right to experience suffering and madness.

Fortunately, the band of pioneers grows a little bit bigger each year. This is how I made the acquaintance of Olivier Jacqmot, whom we now invite to every session of our degree course. Olivier is assistant professor in anatomy at Brussels University and has developed a rare skill in tractography.[11] This is a complicated technology, but in layman's terms it is a branch of cerebral imaging that allows us to visualize the circuits inside the brain. In human beings, this has produced some splendidly sharp images that enable us to show the relationships between different zones and to make visible, in a sense, the support of the unconscious, which has set off a number of arguments around the Freudian unconscious and the cognitive unconscious and whether they are the same.[12]

Reading these various reflections and the work of Olivier Jacqmot, two thoughts come to mind. The first, whether animals can be conscious, is fairly general, but it opens up a wide field of possibility relative to animal consciousness as it applies to cats. The second is specific to the object of our study in that it concerns a fortuitous discovery that tractography has made concerning cats.

A Detour into Consciousness

The idea of a consciousness or cognition in animals has greatly perturbed scientists, philosophers, and religious thinkers alike. Animals, that is, as opposed to humans—I usually say "other animals," but this does not go down well with those who claim animals have no consciousness, either of themselves or of their history or their environment: they are the object of instincts and programmed behavior so they can be represented, as they were in Cartesian theory, as machines without emotions or affect. It should be obvious, then, that without consciousness these animals are merely the playthings of their unconscious, of thoughts generated without their knowledge. I think it is when I address audiences of psychiatrists in human medicine on the theme of the animal psyche that I meet the most resistance, and if I receive a cutting remark or a waspish question, I can usually guarantee that it emanates from a practitioner of one of the more rigorous schools of psychoanalysis. I don't mean to tar all psychoanalysts with the same brush—I was welcomed with great benevolence and curiosity by Gérard Ostermann, for example, with whom I have had impassioned exchanges—but according to them, these poor "animals" have neither consciousness nor an unconscious, which can only be revealed by the psychoanalytic talking cure. These representations mean that we live alongside these "animals" without looking at them and without seeing the evidence of their emotions, their thoughts, their anticipation, their strategies, their individuality, and their suffering, everything that allows you to say that an individual has a psychological life of their own.

As is often the case, this knowledge was at first vulgar in the strict sense of the word—that is, naive and anecdotal—and the evidence is sometimes difficult to demonstrate in a totally rigorous scientific way. We don't have space here to explore all the various proofs of consciousness, but to get back to our domestic cats, consider the following six elements—memory, sentience, language, metacognition, theory of mind, and self-consciousness—and ask yourself whether you would attribute the existence of such a consciousness to Minou, Styx, or Flora.

The Six Criteria of Consciousness

Memory: We have already seen the degree to which bad experiences, which can generate phobic states through the process of heightened sensitivity, always important to prey, condition the psychological life of cats. My image of the red notebook in which they keep a record of everything unpleasant that happens to them is a metaphor of their conscious and unconscious memory.

Sentience: This is the capacity to perceive and sense your environment and to have subjective experiences. If you have two or more cats or even if you compare your cat to itself, you will realize that their sensory perception is filtered to give a subjective and individual representation. In other words, while Mr. Black and Mr. White may live in the same environment, they will not share the same experience at all. Nowadays we attribute such sentience to many representatives of the animal kingdom, and even some from the vegetable kingdom. I don't much like the word: I know that, for many, it is a way of advancing a notion of at the very least a minimal consciousness in animals, but I find it merely strengthens the barrier that it endeavors to break down: humans have consciousness, animals have sentience. It seems much more fruitful to me to accord consciousness to all, as it is in any case not the same consciousness.

Every species in its Umwelt is different, and each individual in that species is unique, even if the area of common ground is more extensive the nearer two individuals are on the tree of evolution. I find it much easier to imagine the world of a chimpanzee or a dog than that of a cat, whose behavioral repertoire is further from ours as a species. But what about the representation of a fish? Some scientists have established proof of pain in these species and opened the door to a minimal animal consciousness.[13]

Language: Though not on the level of articulated language, many animals have complex structures of communication that constitute protolanguages. In cats, no fewer than twenty-one different types of vocalization have been described, studied, and classified, and that was in two recent articles, not just in classic studies in feline ethology.[14] Human companions of cats are generally familiar with every sound their cat emits, from threats to requests for contact. A dictionary might define language primarily as communication between humans, but will also define it as any system of signs allowing communication; in cats this involves both sounds and the use of pheromones, which constitute a subtle form of language.

Metacognition: This is the animal's capacity to know that it does or doesn't know something. There have been studies made on dogs, notably by the Hungarian ethologist Ádám Miklósi and colleagues, and on rats. While there have been no comparable studies on cats, you only need to see them sizing up a leap before doing it to realize that they have a clear consciousness of what they can and can't do.

Theory of Mind: Despite the name, there is no theory involved, just the capacity to attribute to another individual, of the same species or not, a mental state that cannot be observed, such as an intention or desire, for example. This attribution of intention can be seen all the time in the wild, in the predator-prey relationship, which is much less straightforward than we might originally think. Sometimes prey and predator can stand at a water hole just a few yards apart when it is time for drinking and not time for hunting, and at times like this the lack of an intention to hunt can be clearly imputed. As so often happens, behavioral pathology brings this capacity into relief when it is altered or abolished, as in the case of Melly, where the state of derealization distorted the perception of intentions and the cat saw potential hostility in the whole environment.

Self-Consciousness: In some basic research by Gordon Gallup, inspired by the work of the Swiss psychologist Jean Piaget on the stages of child development, many animal species were put forward to do the famous mirror test, which was set up—somewhat prematurely—as an absolute proof of self-consciousness.[15]

These days scientists no longer make this a test of self-recognition. It is easy to see that, even if this test may be applied to a species for whom sight is of major importance, it is of little use for species that predominantly rely on their sense of smell, for example. When you live with a cat, you see over and over again how it pays attention to its appearance, to its grooming, and when you observe its behaviors as a whole, you are left in very little doubt that it has an idea of itself in the world that surrounds it.

*   *   *

If you consider these six criteria, I would be very surprised if you concluded that your cat does not have the characteristics of a conscious being. Not a human consciousness, which is without doubt more elaborate, more symbolic, and has a much superior sense of time, but one involving a perception of its own life, its integrity, and the limits of its environment.

The Curious Split Circuit in the Feline Brain

Olivier Jacqmot pioneered the use of tractography on domestic animals. The first attempts were tricky, whether with dogs or with cats, but little by little he refined the technique and the first results began to appear. The technique has been applied to a very small number of cats: only six have been studied so far. They all presented the same peculiarity: their corpus callosum, the system that allows communication between the two brain hemispheres, seemed to be split in two, a front one and a rear one. We are far from understanding the significance of this anatomical anomaly, still farther from knowing whether it exists in all cats.

If it turns out to be the case for all cats, I see that as an extra confirmation of their double nature, which would require the parallel operation of two circuits: one protecting the integrity of the prey, the other the efficiency of the predator. This unusual brain will no doubt require a lot of time to map, decipher, and understand. As of today, it piques our interest and commands our respect; given its diversity and complexity, it's easy to imagine that it will be prone to dysfunctions that we are only just beginning to understand. Perhaps we need to come up with a very different type of psychiatry that integrates the possibility of suffering in one or the other circuit? Could the states of derealization concern only one of these two "brains"?

This possible duality is already known in dolphins, whose two cerebral hemispheres take turns to sleep so that there is always one that is alert to ensure the minimal movement required to swim and when surfacing to breathe. We have seen the case of Tilikum, the killer whale, who also possessed two quite independent hemispheres. Did his problem arise from just one of these hemispheres or the connection between the two? This opens up vast new fields of research, as Dr. Jacqmot's use of tractography to study cats demonstrates.

For the time being, we are able to describe what we actually observe triggering these states of marked derealization. We already spend too much time rebutting skepticism and sometimes a naive and reductive idealism that won't entertain the possibility of animal mental pathology but makes humans responsible for everything.

The time has come to advance along the road of science: we owe it to cats, now our companions of choice, to give them the care they deserve. We must improve our knowledge, establish solid proofs and reference points, forget our preconceptions about humans and other species, and put our medicine at their service. Psychiatric vets try to do that on a day-to-day basis, but we need everyone—pioneers like Olivier Jacqmot, veterinary colleges, even the manufacturers of psychotropic medicines—to help build the whole theoretical corpus that will enable us to go further. When I say that, I measure the distance we have yet to travel in order to promote this discipline, which has well-being as its aim and knowledge as its weapon, and luckily there are more and more people willing to pick up the baton.

In order to fully convince you of the reality of these states of derealization, I now call to the witness stand Hannibal, a house cat who met a tragic fate.

Hannibal: A Story That Ended Badly

This handsome gray-and-white house cat with green eyes might never have come to see me for a consultation, and perhaps that is still the thing that surprises me most.

I was doing research for a TV program on cats with interesting histories. Through word of mouth at one of the veterinary hospitals where I work, I ended up with Hannibal before me on my table. I wasn't very surprised that the reason was trivial: a friend of Véronique, his owner, had apparently stepped on his tail, which provoked in response a bite on the ankle. I already had an idea of what I was going to say in my report: aggressive attacks due to irritation linked to frustration, hunger, or pain; an absence of hierarchy, the importance of heightened sensitivity, respect for the body; the superfluous and fragile aspect of the relationship, even if attachment is at the heart of a kitten's development. Although the visit was set up as part of the program, the consultation itself was not fake. So I listened when Véronique talked and I carried out a normal consultation.

At the same time, I placed the cat carrier on the table and opened the door: Hannibal looked at me and allowed himself to be stroked with an amiable indifference. After a few moments of scratching his chin, I saw the tip of his tail twitch, so I broke off the contact; he licked himself a little at the spot where I had touched him but stayed in the same place (though he was quite at liberty to get out of his carrier and explore the room). I touched him again, and his edginess returned, but I continued—gently—in order to judge his level of tolerance and the intensity of his reaction. This came less than a minute later, and he bit my hand with the same degree of control that I was exerting. I could barely feel the contact of his teeth, and when I stopped stroking, he opened his mouth immediately, freeing my hand, which was unmarked. My first impression was of a well-adapted cat. We needed to dig a bit deeper.

"You said that your friend stepped on his tail?"

"Yes . . . I mean, well, she said she didn't. . . ."

I pricked up my ears.

"Oh? What did she say exactly?"

"That she was on the balcony next to the cat. She sensed that he was staring at her and she said that he lunged at the back of her leg, though I'm not sure that I believe her. But he did wound her badly: he sank his teeth into her and took off a strip of skin."

"Ah yes, not too surprising! Were there other episodes like this?"

"Yes, with her again actually, on another occasion."

"Tell me about it."

"A couple of weeks after this first incident, she came back and we were sitting on the sofa, chatting. Hannibal was walking through the room when he stopped, stared at my friend, and then came toward her. . . . He jumped onto her and bit her on the belly, tearing her T-shirt and taking off another strip of skin, and then went after her arm. He attacked it really hard and bit through cloth, skin, and even part of the muscle."

"Yes, but this is a very different problem from the one we were talking about. These attacks are really strange. . . . Were there any others?"

"Believe it or not, my friend never came back," said Véronique with a smile.

"I'm not surprised. But attacks on other people?"

"Yes, three weeks after this last incident, another friend came to visit. I was suspicious. Hannibal has only shown this behavior with women so far. Suddenly I saw his expression change. I just had time to grab my friend by the arm and drag her out onto the balcony, and Hannibal rushed at us. He attacked the window and seemed to be beside himself. I called my husband on my mobile, and he came along in biking leathers, with boots and gloves, and together we managed to lock Hannibal in another room."

"You must have been very frightened. . . ."

"When it happened, I was mainly thinking about my friend, but after the event it occurred to me that if I had tried to get in the way, he would have gone for me."

We have spoken a lot about the work of empathy with cats, and it is important, but we mustn't forget the emotions of the owners. This scene would have been very shocking for Véronique, not to mention her two friends. Since then, the cat had been locked away anytime a female acquaintance came to the apartment.

We had now wandered a long way from the original premise of the program, but I was gripped by this case, which I could tell was an important one.

I started suggesting that Hannibal had some psychiatric condition and I could sense the resistance in my client, who after all had only wound up here by chance. She'd come here more or less as a favor to us, and here I was talking to her about her cat being mad. That must have been rather disturbing.

I let her mull it over for a while. I was approaching this cautiously not least because I was far from certain in my own mind, even if my assumptions were robust.

After assessing all of Hannibal's principal functions, I had a clinical picture of a cat who was normal except in these aggressive episodes. There was no anxiety involved here, no deficiency of self-control, but nevertheless a state of massive derealization whenever a crisis occurred.

I offered the owner a treatment involving a medication from behavioral therapy. Selegiline—the medication we used on Nougatine—was our first line of attack in these cases, with the awareness that (this was my main theory) if it was a dissociative syndrome, the equivalent in our carnivores of human schizophrenia, it would be barely effective or indeed not work at all.

An adapted behavioral therapy would involve: a close reading of any signals of threat, which might be quite subtle, in order to get to a place of safety; a redirection of the attacks onto acceptable objects; sometimes an attempt at disruption—for example, a squirt from a plant spray bottle.

None of this would work once the crisis was under way and the cat was in a state of "mad" fury: at that point, nothing could stop it. The first of the above measures, then, was really to ensure the safety of visitors, especially female ones, and making sure that they didn't come into contact with Hannibal the cannibal.

We kept in touch with the cat's owner in the months following this consultation. Neither Véronique nor her husband, nor anyone else in fact, bought into the idea that Hannibal might be "mad"; indeed, some of their friends suggested that it might be the vet himself who was suffering from mental illness.

In cases of this kind, I don't argue, I just wait. If I've got it wrong, which happens not infrequently, well, that's good

189

news for the cat. I just prefer to anticipate the worst that might happen. With Hannibal, the recurrence of these crises eventually convinced Véronique that her cat was indeed presenting the symptoms described in the diagnosis.

Then, the treatment: in the beginning there was a fear that the medication I had prescribed for such a serious illness might itself be dangerous and capable of "frazzling the brain" of the unfortunate animal. It was fairly easy for me to offer reassurance on this product: apart from its effectiveness in regulating mood, it is very safe to use and is even good at protecting nerve cells.

Although the product I had prescribed is safe, it is designed for use on dogs, and so the pills are on the large side and it's quite a challenge to get them down a cat's throat. That subsequently proved to be a complication: this time, Hannibal reacted like all cats do. On the first day, giving him the pill wasn't easy; on the second, it was even more complicated; by the third, it had become impossible—all because of this phenomenon of heightened sensitivity.

Véronique complained: Hannibal ran away from her and he was very disturbed; she found him quite nervous. He threatened her husband, though without scratching or biting him; Hannibal seemed afraid of him and would go into the next room.

The couple also had a little calico cat called Lulu. When Hannibal started his treatment and began to change his behavior, Lulu became disturbed and anxious, to the extent that she began licking herself so roughly that she pulled out her fur. Their behaviors were no doubt connected.

Bit by bit, Véronique realized how serious Hannibal's condition was. I received detailed reports: the attacks were fierce enough, but the phases of unexplained terror were also overwhelming. Suddenly, this unfortunate cat was reacting as if he had been subjected to some terrifying sight or smell that he could not escape even by seeking refuge at the back of a cupboard or under the bed.

Sometimes a deceptive calm would wipe away the menace: weeks might pass without any accidents or terrors. Then there would be a new, very worrying episode. Such as the day a female friend arrived and managed to stroke Hannibal, who suddenly gave her a hard stare, and Véronique did not have time to lock him away. One day, it was her mother who was almost attacked, and they were both very afraid. From irrational fears to unpredictable attacks, Hannibal's life and life with Hannibal had become a succession of strong emotions and setbacks.

Véronique and her husband still clung to one faint hope: they lived in an apartment and, like many people, thought that being cooped up there could be partly responsible for the cat's condition. They planned to move and were waiting impatiently for the day to arrive. The first weeks of life with access to the outside for the cat seemed to confirm this: everything seemed so much better, and I received an enthusiastic email. Hannibal accepted anybody and everybody, he even allowed himself to be stroked by people he barely knew, and Lulu also seemed more peaceful. Then, after four weeks of shared pleasure, one day, when Véronique was packing for a trip, she saw Hannibal, with dilated eyes and a furious expression, pounce on poor Lulu, who was so terrorized she peed on him. Emotional micturition is the ultimate physical expression of an intense emotion. Lulu shrieked, and when Véronique tried to get between them, Hannibal attacked her too. She had time only to escape to the balcony, with the cat attacking the window.

That day made her feel so afraid that, together with her husband, they took the "horrible decision," as she wrote to me, to "put Hannibal to sleep."

In cases like this, this is news we always dread to hear but expect almost daily: How can you live with a primed grenade in the house? There is no judgment on my part, just a great sadness, the feeling, however unwarranted, that I have betrayed my medical oath.

Hannibal's was a story that ended badly because we don't yet know enough, our means are limited, and our medicines insufficient to relieve the terrible suffering of these cats who are locked up in their own heads.

My aim in presenting this case to you is to open up a way so that in future there are more of us who are able and willing to care for and alleviate the suffering of these few mad cats. For that to happen we need to make advances in the science of the mental illness of animals—and of cats in particular—and for all medical professionals to play their part in transmitting their knowledge.

5

A Symbol of Our Time

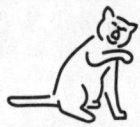

Time spent with a cat is never wasted time.

—*Colette*

To cap off this survey of behavioral pathology and our relationship with cats, it seems important to me to discuss the extent to which our feline companions, usually without realizing it, pose fundamental questions about our relationship with other animals, and sometimes even with other humans. Cats are often called as witnesses in some of the polemics of our time and can give us an offbeat take on things.

To complete this journey of initiation, let's try to answer four questions that take us somewhat away from our main subject but bring us back to our starting point, namely the cat as witness or symbol of our times. Can we still nowadays separate psychological and physical well-being? What is our attitude toward the autonomy of these living creatures for whom we have responsibility, whom we look after and love?

How do we envisage aging, end of life, and the limits of care in ways that are acceptable both for us and for our animal companions? What do cats tell us about changes in our social attitudes toward authority, hierarchy, and education? Let's look at each of these points in turn.

One Health, One Welfare

Our first question, about the connection between psychological and physical well-being, should not need to be asked, but I am well placed to know that there is still a ways to go before all involved—the humans living in contact with their cats, the vets, the breeders—are convinced that there can be no separation between the two. We must also beware of the opposite: of overemphasizing the relationship between body and mind.

There is a gray area between behavioral and organic issues, between the influence of the habitat and the expression of ill-being. The domestic feline species is emblematic of these questions, and the responses of our feline companions are intriguing. For a long time we have defended the concept, now regarded as essential, of "one health," and the extension of that idea is captured by the slogan "One Health, One Welfare."

Fashionable though it may be, the concept does touch upon the interdependence of physical health, behavioral balance, collaboration between species, and integration in a harmonious and protected environment.

Simple Minds

Sometimes, things are much simpler, and cats may display undesirable behavior that is not pathological, indicative of madness, but instead is an attempt to reestablish harmony in their world.

We saw with Choupette that a simple change of litter can alter a cat's very nature: this case shows us how much cats exemplify the idea of "One Health, One Welfare." A house move, the arrival of a baby—these are major changes, and so everyone is aware of their potential impact on feline equilibrium; but while a piece of furniture out of place or a suitcase left in an entrance may appear insignificant, these can be enough to disrupt a cat's emotional balance.

This is the message underlying some of the undesirable behaviors that we have encountered during the course of our guided tour, which can now be understood in the light of the new understanding of cats that we have acquired. While these behaviors can be diagnosed according to the illnesses described earlier (biotopathy, schezipathy, and so on), they can just as easily stand alone, often signifying nothing other than the cat's wish to reestablish balance in its world or the expression of a cultural misinterpretation between them and us.

The Scratching Cat

If your cat scratches something that you value, and it observes you out of the corner of its eye and runs away as soon as you approach to scold it, don't take it the wrong way. Your cat lives with you and knows you better than you know it. It is just doing what it has to do in order to organize its living space, and this behavior is a necessary part of that, but it has learned that you might have a negative reaction and so anticipates it. If you don't punish it in a painful or scary way, this can continue over a long period of time and give you the impression that your cat is mocking you. It is simply trying to align its needs with your strictures. It is not trying to provoke you but rather is trying to walk the narrow path that makes cohabitation possible. If you put yourself in your cat's place, you'll understand what it is trying to do and allow it to do so in a better spot nearby (no point in putting a scratching post at the back of the bathroom; it will not serve any purpose) while making the area you want to protect unsuitable for scratching (see box).

The potential error springs from a misunderstanding: you think that your cat wants to sharpen its claws, and of course cats tend to do this in order to scrape off dead tissue, but this is not the principal motivation behind this behavior. If it was, you would have no problem directing it away from your favorite sofa or armchair: your cat would happily do its scratching somewhere else. But in this case the place is as important as the action itself. As we have seen in the chapter devoted to the living space, making their zone of isolation into a sanctuary is an essential need for many cats.

Don't punish your cat, manage its space, and harmony will be restored.

> ### How to Dissuade Your Cat from Sharpening Its Claws
>
> Strips of transparent double-sided adhesive tape on the scratching place, or a foil blanket, can make the target area uncomfortable for the cat. If at the same time you put a suitable scratching post (for example, one with a rope wrapped around its whole length) at your cat's disposal nearby, this has a very good chance of working.

Taco the Biter

Not all biting is aggressive. In cats it sometimes has to do with pleasure, even passion. Remember Isis, whom we met in chapter 3. The first bites were not intentionally aggressive but occurred while she was being stroked. The biting, which was a sign of excitement, was misinterpreted and led to punishments, which merely aggravated the situation. It is very rare in cats that biting on its own is a manifestation of aggression. More often the biting is accompanied or preceded by threatening behavior: raised paw, flattened ears, even swipes with claws when this is not enough to keep the imagined threat at arm's length. And cats—"normal" cats, at least—tend to avoid conflict rather than provoke it.

That said, I remember Taco, a cat I saw in my consulting room, who was adored by the humans he lived with but who "hated" their neighbor so much that when he spotted him, he would slip under the fence and advance on him in a menacing manner, even though the man was on his own property. If this threat didn't work and since the neighbor had often retaliated to defend his territory, Taco would rush at him and bite him hard on the calf if he managed to catch him. The whole neighborhood was up in arms about this, and a petition was raised and sent to the local council, who took the matter seriously. This was a case where we were not able to put a treatment in place; instead, Taco's owners chose to send him to live in the country with a relative of theirs, who had several hectares of land. That was no guarantee that some other neighbor didn't end up subjected to the wrath of this cat, who couldn't tolerate any opposition.

More often, in cases of isolated biting, we have to look for reasons other than aggression to understand the behavior: unrestrained play, pleasurable overstimulation, a response to excitation. Biting, while painful and shocking for the human on the receiving end of it, is not always what it seems.

Dirty Danae

Let us recall that, because the harmony of their living space is of paramount importance, cats may, as a result of minor incidents, lose what many consider to be an unchangeable characteristic of their species: their cleanliness, the fact that they do their business in litter boxes or outside the house. As we saw with Choupette and others, the first key task when this happens is to establish whether this is due to disposal or marking behavior.

Danae was a female cat who seemed relaxed, and yet she had been marking with urine almost daily for a month. There appeared to have been little to disrupt her: a new table in the entrance hall, friends coming over a couple of times for a meal with her owners. Danae started marking and was scolded, though not especially severely. While she seemed very stable, she was marking and showing signs of a depressive state, although this could not yet be diagnosed with any degree of certainty. We were already at the point where there were some signs, but not enough to establish a diagnosis. I had to explain and decode the cat's behavior, endeavoring to open wide the doors of her mind to show everyone that there was no malice in her behavior, just suffering. Danae was able to recover her balance within a few weeks, but for every cat who comes in for a consultation, or rather whose owners bring it in for one, how many others sink into a state of chronic depression left untreated?

These are quite straightforward behavioral changes, which can be reversed in a matter of days or weeks, and are fairly classic sources of complaint by exasperated owners—understandably so. But cats are also very good at demonstrating the close links between psychological well-being and physical health. They remind us, like neuroscientist Antonio Damasio, not to make Descartes's error and see the mind and body as separate.[1] Emotions influence our physical organism, and things that happen in the body have significant reper-cussions on our inner life.

Moon, the Cat Who Tore His Fur Out

One case made a deep impression on me and led to changes in our practice. It happened twenty years ago and concerned Moon, a sweet, gentle cat who devoted abnormal attention to his grooming and pulled his fur out. We saw in the case of Melly that this can be a sign of a serious psychiatric illness, but that is not the most common explanation. In the vast majority of cases, it signifies a permanent and inhibited anxious state. Vets see a lot of cats that are overweight and no longer have any fur on their bellies. Generally, the advice to the owners is to help the animal to lose weight, but there is still not enough emphasis on the link between two classic manifestations of anxiety: compulsive licking and binge eating.

Sometimes even owners are surprised to see this large area of the belly without fur. Cats lick themselves in silence and there is no reason why people living with cats should be aware of the loss of fur. This extensive feline alopecia, as we have seen earlier, has many causes (including fleas—don't forget the fleas!), but its symmetrical position on the belly, sometimes extending to the insides of the two thighs, suggests compulsive licking triggered by anxiety.

With Moon, it was rather different: he didn't lick himself in the privacy of his zone of isolation and he didn't do it at night when his human companions were asleep. He did it all the time: he would grab tufts of fur on his side, tug them with all his strength, and yank them out. He even did it during the consultation, which is rare. Cats may be inhibited, aggressive, or calm during consultations, but in my experience none of them feel sufficiently at ease to consider my exam room as a zone of isolation offering them the security to express a behavior that renders them vulnerable. I watched Moon pulling out his fur, frankly surprised that he had so much left, and I started to investigate. I looked for all the causes we have examined together that can alter a cat's emotional balance. His living space was well set up, there were no issues with the frequency of his meals, his zones of disposal were identifiable and stable. Once it has been established that there is no external cause of the imbalance, we have to remember that anxiety can also be rooted internally. We didn't find any parasites either on or inside Moon.

Following a hunch, I checked his viral status with the referring colleague with whom I run my consultations. The cat was vaccinated against feline leukemia, but what about FIV (feline immunodeficiency virus)? FIV is a virus from the same family as HIV, even though—and I can't emphasize this strongly enough—there is absolutely no connection between them and no cross-contamination. It weakens the immune defenses and exposes the cat to infection, though the clinical descriptions rarely cite behavioral modifications. The clinical picture didn't have much to offer—compulsive licking is not described in this illness, but since it affected general balance, it was worth checking. One quick blood test later and the result was clear: Moon was indeed infected with FIV. We had to be careful not to make too instant an association between this infection and the clinical signs, but at least his abnormal behavior had allowed us to detect it, to take charge of it and adopt measures to prevent further contamination. Moon, like so many other cats, was living proof that behavioral balance cannot be properly assessed without an exhaustive appreciation of the physical state, and it is necessary to see the big picture as well as the detail in order to perform a good behavioral consultation. It is the role of vets to increase their knowledge and add behavioral changes as a new string to their diagnostic bow.

Behavioral Issues and Infections

Few articles in scientific journals have explored the connection between behavioral issues and infection. There are occasional references to mood problems and aggressivity, but no in-depth consideration of behavioral semiology.

I've found one article on the link between infection and behavior, but in experimental conditions with an intravenous injection of a high dose of the virus on six eight-week-old kittens.[2] In real life, contamination usually occurs between adults, through biting or sexual contact. The study showed a learning deficiency in all six cats, with lower-quality memorization (more mistakes made in simple tests for spatial recognition and finding food, involving failing to return to a place already explored). In the wild, this type of "forgetfulness" could cost a cat dearly, if the area they revisited harbored a predator.

One of our students started researching the repercussions of FIV infection on behavior. He studied thirty cats infected with FIV and compared them to thirty cats that had tested negative but presented symptoms that could evoke this illness.[3] That was a good sample. The results were clear: the cats infected with FIV presented more behavioral issues than the uninfected cats. There were more problems with uncleanliness but also more cognitive problems, which confirmed the experimental data. Remarkably, infected cats dreamed less. We saw earlier how important dreaming is, especially to our domestic felines, whose double nature requires even more ordering of day-to-day events, a sorting process that is rendered possible by dream work. This explains at least in part the unstable moods in FIV-positive cats and the occurrence of unpredictable aggressive episodes that the owners cannot account for.

Moon had shown me the way, and this new research confirmed that it is a mistake not to consider individual cats as a whole.

Kita, and Her Intermittent Suffering

Cats are prone to very painful episodes of cystitis. This inflammation of the bladder creates a pressing need to pee, though sometimes with very little urine to expel. Every time a cat urinates it is painful, and sometimes there is blood. I remember

Kita from my years in general practice. Before I became a vet psychiatrist, I worked for fifteen years as a regular vet, seeing dogs and cats in my clinic in Toulon. I was already interested in cat behavior and I was very sensitive to the suffering of Kita, a small female Siamese, and the way in which she expressed it. Two or three times a year, Kita suffered episodes of cystitis, and her owner immediately knew when it was happening: normally very clean, this little cat would squat in the sink or bathroom and emit a few drops of urine flecked with blood as if to warn her mistress. I've subsequently heard this behavior described too often by too many owners to think that it is merely fortuitous. A message? Definitely. A way of asking for help? Very likely.

When we run analyses, they are often disappointing, revealing sterile urine without bacteria, the signature of an infection, but with an absence of kidney stones or crystals. That is why this cystitis is called idiopathic, to emphasize that the cause is unknown. All treatments work, but not applying treatment and just being patient also works. The challenge is not to seek an immediate cure for the infection, which lasts a few days before it normally sorts itself out of its own accord, but to space out the episodes over the course of the year.

This is where Tony Buffington, an American veterinary doctor formerly at Ohio State University and now at the University of California, Davis, comes into the picture. He revolutionized the small world of internal veterinary medicine when he claimed that cystitis was also the consequence of anxiety pheromones and that it was necessary to take into consideration the stressful events in the cat's life, especially those occurring during its period of development.[4] I believe that this changed the minds of many of my colleagues who had hitherto taken no interest whatsoever in the psychological health of their feline patients.

Tony Buffington and his team put forth the theory that since the causes of idiopathic cystitis include stress, then the care could not be purely medical but must at the very least take the cat's habitat into account. Buffington formulated a method of multimodal modification of the environment and showed that it was more effective than classical treatment based on antibiotics and bladder protectors.[5]

Eventually, this will pave the way for a holistic approach to medical treatment. In a recent article in which he reviewed his twenty years of research, Buffington took a global view, citing genetic research in psychiatry but—and this remains a painful mystery to me—without making any link with feline psychiatry.[6] He chose instead to focus on the balance between the central system for stress response and the control system, and he even coined a new term, "Pandora syndrome," to encompass all the causes that can lead to symptoms of idiopathic cystitis.[7]

I am very grateful to Buffington for his work, which has allowed us to place the uniqueness of the individual, the links between environment and health, between stress and physical illness, at the center of veterinary medicine. However, it is a matter of huge regret to me that he didn't progress from that to a complete vision of domestic felines that included the possibility of suffering, of mental illness—in short, psychiatry. Yet this article, which is a summary of years of research by a clinical professor of medicine at the University of California, Davis, School of Veterinary Medicine, is coauthored by a professor of behavioral medicine.

In North America, the term "veterinary psychiatry" is still considered scary. This is beginning to change with the new generation of practitioners. A few years ago, an American colleague, Dr. Lisa Radosta, presented a paper at the World Small Animal Veterinary Association (WSAVA) entitled "Veterinary Psychiatry Potpourri," while another colleague, Sagi Denenberg—a Slovak who studied in his home country, then in Israel and Canada, a member of the American College of Veterinary Behaviorists and the European College of Animal Welfare and Behavioural Medicine—published a book in 2020 entitled *Small Animal Veterinary Psychiatry*, which finally used the word "psychiatry," anchoring our discipline in a medical approach.[8]

I have no doubt that once those who refuse to see the evidence have retired, veterinary psychiatry will become established globally and our American colleagues will come back to tell us how important it is. What counts at the end of the day is that other animals, particularly those with whom we share our habitat, should be seen as a whole: we should look at both their physical health, which vets have been taking care of for a long time, and their mental balance, whose importance we are just starting to recognize but which will in due course lead to the best form of care.

This handful of examples of behavior that is undesirable but not always a sign of pathology and these two examples of a global form of medicine—the first combining virology and behavioral medicine, the other urology and psychiatry—shows us that the increased presence of cats in our veterinary clinics has compelled us to pay more attention to the ideas of global medicine.

Pain, a feeling of weakness, a disproportionate fear, and the whole subtle balance can be disrupted, and life can become complicated. Cats remind us that a happy life is a fragile thing that deserves our full attention.

A Cat's Right to Choose

Cats are also a symbol of well-being and are often called as witnesses in polemical arguments. As we look at some of these, we will see that cats are frequently embroiled in controversy but little account is taken of their view of things. For example, do we have the right to impose on them a life without access to the outside? Is it ethical to perform systematic sterilization when all research on well-being demonstrates the importance of sexuality in the flourishing of an individual?

Hector Doesn't Like Going Outside

Hector was very important to the couple who brought him in to see me. They were desperate, yet Hector appeared to be doing well—at least he wasn't doing badly—but let's hear what Rebecca had to say.

"We used to live in an apartment with Hector, but that didn't fit with our values. We wanted to offer our cat the best, and we thought it was very important that he could go outside. Besides, it was a lifestyle choice for us too: we wanted to have an outdoor space for ourselves, to be more in contact with nature. The first time Hector went outside, not very far, we accompanied him. He then went out on his own but instantly shot back inside as if he'd seen the devil himself. After that, he never went out again."

"But you left the door open?"

"Of course, once spring arrived. . . . He sits on the front steps and maybe takes a few tentative steps outside, but then dashes back inside again. He doesn't make use of the garden at all."

"Understood. We will look at Hector's behavioral balance and see how he is doing."

In this situation, with my psychiatrist vet's hat on, I have a list of points to consider. Firstly, is the animal well? Are his needs satisfied? Is there a way to diminish the disappointment of the humans who accompany the cat by enabling the missing behavior, in this case going out into the garden?

My focus as a vet is always on the animal, and that is how it should be, but it seems worthwhile to recall that our role is to care for the humans too, to diminish their suffering and help them live a harmonious life with their pet.

In the course of our consultations, while exploring all the cat's behaviors, we might change direction when it becomes possible to trace a line between undesirable but normal behavior and a pathological state. That is why we do not limit ourselves—sometimes to the surprise of the animals' owners—to their original reason for bringing the cat in. If there is, for example, an anxious state, there is a good chance that we will be able to detect its effects upon the animal's sleep, appetite, contact with its own body, and exploratory habits. We have to observe everything, question everything, to obtain a clear, well-rounded picture and arrive at a precise diagnosis.

In the case of Hector, we had to differentiate between a phobic state that prevented him from adapting and a normal attitude of prudence in relation to an environment any cat would find threatening. The semiological inquiry revealed nothing abnormal: Hector seemed fine in himself and appeared simply to have decided to limit his life to the interior of the house. No doubt his development had predisposed him to choose this option, and the unpleasant experience of his second excursion outdoors had merely confirmed his decision, but there was no need to treat him.

Rebecca was relieved, as was Thomas, her partner, to learn that Hector was doing fine and that he was well-balanced. But they also felt a keen disappointment:

"All the same, he doesn't make use of the garden. . . ."

"That's his choice for the time being. When you bump into the Terminator at a bend in the path, you're not in a hurry to repeat the experience. . . ."

I gave them my explanation about the little red book, the prey–predator duality, the importance of a heightened sensitivity, and the need for patience. Hector might one day decide to give exploring the outdoors another go . . . or maybe not. In any case, the rest of his behaviors—the games he shared with them, the hunts after mice and lizards that wandered inside the house, his shared zone of isolation, his consistent and meticulous use of the litter box, his regular but well-regulated appetite, his frequent facial marking of places around the house and on them—all this indicated a well-balanced cat with a full and varied behavioral repertoire.

We came up with some strategies to lure Hector outside and allow him to have a good time without ever forcing him. I would hear back from them a year later. Rebecca and Thomas discovered a short time after the consultation that there was a more or less feral cat who frightened all the house cats in the neighborhood. They stroked Hector and played with him outside, but he remained true to himself and led a happy and harmonious life as an indoor cat.

Hector provides us with one response to that polemical view that stigmatizes owners who offer their cat only a life indoors. Sometimes the cat itself chooses to stay inside a reassuring space that offers them everything they need for their well-being.

Émile Zola wrote a novella on this theme, telling the story of an Angora cat who wants to experience the freedom of alley cats but, after a night of horror and hostile encounters with other cats, in the rain, unable to find anything to eat, chooses to return to where it knows it can find comfort and be well fed.[9]

A Field Survey

In order to obtain more substantial scientific evidence, one of our students, as mentioned earlier, researched the living conditions, the behavioral repertoire, and the prevalence of behavioral issues in cats who went out and those without access to the outside.[10]

It was a large trial: 351 cats were included in the study, which provided a lot of information and one major lesson. There are no more behavioral issues (in particular regarding the two main complaints, uncleanliness and aggression) among confined cats than there are among cats who have access to the outside. And the cats purr just as much, whether they live inside or out.

Of course, some differences did emerge from this survey: more often, cats who didn't go out manifested those "fifteen minutes of madness," bouts of agitated dashing about than cats who went out, and they were more likely to indulge in episodes of simulated predation. In the same vein, and this seems logical, the cats who lived in an apartment or a house without going out engaged in more phases of play than those who enjoyed other activities outdoors.

These differences make perfect sense: behavior as fundamental as predation either is expressed "for real" on natural prey or requires some other outlet that allows cats to satisfy this need. Play, a juvenile trait that continues into adulthood if ever there was one, is expressed much more in a protected environment, where there is little fear of being in a situation of mortal risk, than outside, where constant vigilance is required. The difference in biotope involves a variation in the behavioral repertoire, which isn't surprising.

What we were looking for was the answer to the main question: Does living without access to the outside create more behavioral issues? Is there any proof that confinement generates unhappiness and increases the prevalence of behavioral pathology?

Of course, a single study does not provide a definitive answer, but it was a large sample, and the distribution was homogeneous, which does mean we can legitimately draw certain conclusions.

First of all, it seems obvious that the severe psychiatric illnesses that we have discussed—bipolar dysthymia or dissociative syndrome—are not caused by the environment. Furthermore, they are rare and are not associated more with one set of living conditions than with another. What is interesting is that the aim of this survey was to check whether the symptoms that might lead to an anxious state are more common in confined cats. It would then be legitimate—in fact almost obligatory—to recommend possible access to the outdoors for each cat.

But on every point that can act as an indicator of an anxious state, we found no significant differences relating to living place. Rolling skin syndrome (RSS) is not more common in indoor cats. When there are no fleas, we know that this is a classic sign of a pathological, phobic, or anxious state.

Irritation attacks are major symptoms of an active, intermittent anxious state. In the event that confinement generates frustration and imbalance, we should expect to see an increase in aggressive episodes. This is not the case. If living conditions can generate a permanent, inhibited anxious state, then we should find displacement activities such as compulsive licking leading to ventral alopecia (loss of fur on the belly). This is not the case either.

Finally, as Choupette and many other cats have demonstrated, the difficulty of structuring their living space if it does not comply with their requirements often triggers either undesirable disposal or marking. We should have found greater uncleanliness among confined cats, but this is not the case.

These results are important given that there are some who would like to blame owners who don't have the possibility of letting their cats go out, even going so far as to strongly advise such people not to get a cat in the first place. These views have no scientific basis and there is no reason for such advice.

Of course, you need to make sure that the indoor cat can satisfy all its needs: that it can explore in three dimensions, have toys to practice hunting, and be able to construct its living space with zones of isolation, feeding, disposal, activity, and varied and well-organized interaction. If all that is in place, there is no justification for disapproval by others.

The Risk of Going to Extremes

A former client called me recently. Having lost his dog, he wanted to get a cat. Wishing to do this in a responsible way, he went online to look for advice. A few days later, he contacted me, distraught: "I'd like to have your advice . . . I've read so much stuff and feel a bit lost. According to some people, if I can't or won't let my cat go out, I am mistreating it, and according to others, if I do let it out, I am creating a danger for other animals. For the time being I've decided to postpone my decision to get a cat. . . ."

We had a good, long chat about this. I told him what I have outlined earlier, that the risk to biodiversity has been exaggerated, that it is possible to equip an outdoor cat with a bell to warn potential prey or fit guards around trees in the vicinity of its home that prevent it from climbing them to get at birds' nests. I also made the point that it is possible to ensure optimal well-being for a cat that can't go out by taking certain measures. Of course, you have to choose a cat or kitten whose developmental background corresponds to its future environment: it will be more difficult for it to adapt to an enclosed space if it has passed the first three months of its life in total freedom and is suspicious of humans. If you know all the requirements of a cat's biotope, the distribution of zones, the marking out of paths, you can tick all the boxes and ensure a varied and harmonious life for your cat.

This matter of being able to go out is, as we have seen, more of a philosophical or ethical bone of contention than based on science. You can't ask science questions for which it doesn't have the answers. Cats constantly demonstrate their capacity to adapt to very different environments. When certain conditions are unacceptable (for example, being forced to live with too many other cats without being able to escape, whether that is in an apartment with 10 other cats or in a refuge with 150), then we will see symptoms of an anxious or depressive state: increased aggression, withdrawal, lack of grooming, uncleanliness, and so on. We are not talking about that, but about situations that allow a cat to be emotionally well-balanced: without going out but with enough stimulation indoors, or by going outside in a controlled manner, whether with its owners opening the door for it or via an electronic cat flap, or cats who mostly live outside with very restricted access indoors. It becomes clear, then, that this tells us much more about what humans believe than about cats themselves.

In this never-ending discussion I think, as always, that the simplest thing is to ask the opinion of the interested parties. I have shared my life with many cats. When I was a student, the cat who lived with us had no access to the outside at all, except during vacations. Minou was a model cat. Well-behaved and knowing where to draw the line, he liked to play with the dog, with whom he got along famously: he had fashioned a little nipple of fur near the dog's neck and around dusk he liked to suck on it and knead it for a few minutes. During the summer vacation we were sometimes in the country, at my house near Toulon, and he was free to come and go as he pleased. Never more than a few dozen yards from the house, but he seemed to appreciate it. Sometimes we would hear a catfight and we would worry, but then we would find him on the windowsill listening to those bad boys going at it hammer and tongs. When the time came to leave, he made us look for him for several minutes. We would find him under a bush or a thicket, in no hurry to return home, but, once discovered, he would slip happily into his carrier to be taken back to the apartment and his games with the dog without showing any physical symptoms or signs of distress.

After him, all the cats I've had have lived in semi-freedom with access to the outdoors on demand, except at night of course, and all shared our life. This is the answer given by millions of cats to those who deplore the fact that pets should be kept captive and subjected to some kind of forced cohabitation. Of course, there are cats who are given no choice in the matter, but, as we have already seen, it is possible to construct a more than satisfactory indoor home.

Sometimes I see cats who express their wish to go out more and who live in conditions that would allow it, but their human companions are too afraid for them to let them out. This makes me think about Clémentine, the mother of the twins in Boris Vian's novel *Heartsnatcher*, who tries to protect them at all cost by chopping down the tree in the garden or locking them up in a cage without walls.[11] But the children eat blue slugs that give them the power to fly and to escape the suffocating worries of their mother. Because my work with humans and with cats relies on empathy, I do not pass judgment. I understand the desire to be protective and I understand the need for freedom. When the cats brought to me seem to ask me for it, when I hear of multiple attempts to gain access to the outside or when their apparent resignation is accompanied by symptoms of pathological inhibition, I advocate on their behalf for permission to go out if I think that is the right answer. Electronic cat flaps and lightweight GPS collars are a good solution—they allow the cat to satisfy its thirst for discovery and the owner to keep a protective eye on it.

When, for one reason or another, that is not possible, I make sure that the cat has everything it needs in its living space so that it can thrive. If you want to live with a cat, don't hesitate; whatever your lifestyle, you will find one who is willing to share it with pleasure. Once again, pay no heed to those descriptions of breeds that promise you a Ragdoll will always behave like its name suggests or that a Persian is made for the indoor life. Match your future cat and its history to the biotope that you can offer it, check that the important criteria are all in place, and get ready for the start of a beautiful friendship.

Cat on a Hot Tin Roof

Once you have negotiated that step, you very soon face another controversial question: Should you neuter your feline companion or not?

For some, the question does not even arise: there is only one rule, and that is compulsory spaying or neutering, sometimes from a very young age. We have seen a plethora of publications recommending ovariectomy (removal of the ovaries) from the age of three months or even earlier.[12] Nowadays we seem to be heading toward something a little more reasonable, and some articles have pointed out the risk of increased anxiety due to raised levels of the luteinizing hormone (LH), rendering cats more susceptible to anxious states.[13] Surgical sterilization cuts off the return of sex hormones to the pituitary gland and hypothalamus, leading to abnormally high levels of LH within the body. Since receptors of this hormone exist in numerous tissues, some question the effect of these raised doses (for example, up to thirty times the normal dose for a neutered cat compared to an "intact" cat) on behavior, since there are receptors in the thyroid, the adrenal glands, and the digestive tract, which we know can modulate emotions and, in the case of the digestive tract, act as a second brain.[14] Although this research was done on dogs, it is hard to believe, despite knowing that cats are different, that it would have no effect on their behavior.

The English-language literature on the subject is not especially interested in depression—this is reserved for human beings, since "dark thoughts" are difficult to prove in other animals. Nonetheless, we regularly encounter depressive states in cats, whether this is a case of acute, posttraumatic anxiety, for example, after some physical punishment, or, more frequently, chronic depression as a result of years of untreated anxiety. It seems that sterilization—especially when performed on very young cats—may contribute to depression. We are familiar with this effect on adult cats who are neutered too late, at the age of six or seven, for example. The abolition of sexual motivation sometimes induces a collapse of activity.

While this should give food for thought to any owner facing this decision, it does not run counter to the necessary control of the stray cat population. The discussion can often get bogged down when these two distinct issues become confused. Everyone claims they are acting for the general good, but they aren't talking about the same thing. As I have already mentioned,[15] cat protection charities have taken up a radical position on this: all cats should be spayed or neutered, in their view, and owners should be prevented from allowing their cat to reproduce. All such initiatives designed to make owners more responsible, as well as initiatives carried out as a partnership between public authorities and animal charities, including a proposed multi-party agreement in France with the aim of managing the stray cat population, are excellent and a step in the right direction. This does not prevent us from considering each cat on its own individual terms.

Pleasure

Specialists in well-being have moved on a lot since those early definitions based on the five freedoms mentioned earlier; nowadays, they define specific zones and take into account the subjective experience of the animal.[16] For example, the food made available may well correspond to all modern dietary requirements, but do the animals derive any real pleasure from eating it? Such notions are based on a new definition of well-being proposed by ANSES (the French National Agency for Health Security),[17] the touchstone for these sorts of reflections in France. It reads as follows: "An animal's well-being is a positive mental and physical state linked to the satisfaction of its physiological and behavioral needs, as well as of its expectations. This state varies according to how the animal itself perceives its situation."

This definition changes the terms of reference: by taking on board behavioral needs and expectations, it makes the animal the real subject of its own existence. By insisting on the importance of the animal's own perception of its situation, it also confirms that well-being is an individual affair above all and that the same life conditions could suit one animal but create a lot of stress, or even an anxious state, in another. There is an individual decision to be made for each cat in relation to its environment, the capacity for control on the part of the humans who live with it, and the consequences of its access to reproduction. There is a difference between letting your tomcat run free, so that he can mate with several females and run the risk of being contaminated with FIV, against which he can't be protected, and taking the decision to allow Princess to have a litter, with a more or less selected male, with kittens that will be cherished and carefully placed with responsible families.

Beyond all these questions lies the issue of pleasure. This new way of envisaging well-being includes sexual satisfaction as a factor. Which raises the question: What do we know about the sexual pleasure of our domestic felines?

The common idiom "like a cat in heat" says more about the expression of desire than about pleasure. These periods can give rise to spectacular manifestations, so much so that sometimes they can lead to a consultation in which people who have never witnessed a cat in heat think that their little female is suffering. She caterwauls, she rubs herself against the wall; her voice has changed, it's more raucous. Let us remember that this species is characterized by provoked ovulation, triggered by mounting, which explains their very high reproductive success rate. The heat does not relent until there is mounting by the male: veterinary students know this and sometimes simulate a mounting with a cotton swab in order to continue studying in peace. But does all this desire lead to pleasure? We know very little about this in the case of female cats. We have very little doubt that female dogs, monkeys, dolphins, and many others experience sexual pleasure, but in female cats it seems very unlikely.

Strong desire, yes, pleasure later through motherhood, contact with the kittens, attachments, as we have demonstrated elsewhere,[18] no doubt about that; but when it comes to sexual pleasure, no sign of it: if anything, the opposite might be true.

As cats are essentially not a social species, we are not surprised to find that there is no amorous display, no flirtation, no seduction. The female is ready, she rolls on the ground, she displays willing acquiescence (if you touch the base of the tail from one side, she will move it to the other side, freeing up access to the vulva). After the male has pursued her for a few minutes, he jumps on top of her and grabs her by the scruff of the neck, biting hard. This causes a lordosis (arching), which facilitates penetration. The penis of the uncastrated male cat has spikes on it, like small thorns on the glans, which make penetration painful and cause the female to howl. Usually this lasts no longer than thirty seconds.

Such speed (the time the two participants are engaged in the act is very short) and efficiency (provoked ovulation) work well for a species for whom security is a number one priority. This doesn't allow any time for pleasure, at least for the female. One explanation was proposed by Thierry Lodé during a teaching assignment on this topic in our veterinary psychiatry course. A professor of the ecology of evolution at the University of Rennes, he is a specialist in animal sexuality.[19]

Having astounded us with the revelation that a female rainbow trout can fake "pleasure" in order to get rid of an overinsistent male, he made the point that in this "war of the sexes" there is an evolutionary advantage for males to try to provoke fidelity on the part of the female. There are only two ways to do this: give her lots of pleasure or hurt her. The reproductive organs of certain males, in particular certain birds, are equipped with hooks that make you wonder what pain they must inflict, and it seems to us that something similar must be going on with the cat species as well. While the characteristics of the mounting meet the requirements of security, they do not allow females to experience pleasure, so that just leaves pain. While we need to tread carefully— this is only a hypothesis after all—this gives at least a partial response to the perception of sexuality in female cats. I am convinced that they derive much pleasure from their kittens, but I think they do not derive pleasure from the sexual act, except insofar as it provides release from a torturous desire.

This is what cats might say to us concerning their freedom: freedom to come and go, freedom of access to a sexuality. Once again, they wrong-foot us and force us not to project our own human feelings and representations onto their lives as pet cats. If we wish to ensure their maximum well-being, they force us to put ourselves in their place, with their biology, their physiology, their nature, their representations of themselves and of the world around them, without us imposing on them our well-meaning desires, our projections of our own fantasies about them or our way of mixing up species without respecting their specificity.

When we speak about the unity of all living creatures, when we speak of ourselves and other animals, this is not to say that we all experience the world in the same way, that our values are universal and should be applied to all species. What we should be reflecting on is our relationship with the autonomy of the living creatures that we have responsibility for, take care of, and love: to what extent we can seek their advice, by observing and understanding their behavior, and take it into account so that we may live together in harmony.

Beyond This Limit

Advances in veterinary medicine are today allowing our feline companions to live to a considerable age and are pushing back the frontiers of what we can do in terms of surgery and other medical treatment.

Cats are very good at asking us almost unanswerable questions and they do it unawares. Their natural capacity for resistance magnified by the help of technology and advances in medicine create problems that don't pose themselves in the same way for humans but are relevant to us too.

How should we—our pets and ourselves—grow old? What degree of degradation is acceptable and to what extent do we wish to maintain the physical function of our bodies while undergoing a major alteration in our cognitive capacities? What message does our pets' old age send us and how do we tolerate it? What are the limits of care we envisage for our pets? Who can say that how you care for a cat is unacceptable? And how should we think about the end of life? Must it always be natural, or can it be assisted, and, in that case, who makes that decision? When science can prevent you from dying but can't always allow you to live, how do we arbitrate?

Usually cats grow old gracefully. These days, as the number of human centenarians increases, it is likewise not unusual for cats to live past twenty, which raises the issue of feline old age. Improved living conditions, ongoing protection, and medical progress have put a brake on time for human beings and other animals. They have enabled a longevity that just does not exist in the natural world. With cats now growing much older than they would if left to their own devices in the wild, what does this tell us?

Statistics, particularly those derived from studies at the University of California, Davis, indicate a very different life expectancy between indoor cats, which tend to manage between ten and fifteen years, and cats who live outdoors, whose life expectancy can be as low as two to four years. This might seem to suggest, somewhat bizarrely, that for the sake of your cat's health you should not let it go out because of the risk of drastically shortening its life.[20] We should not confuse cats that are able to go out from time to time with ones who live in the wild. Nearly all of my cats went out, except for those who didn't want to, and almost all of them lived for more than ten years.

Of course, a cat that goes out is more prone to the hazards of road traffic or to viruses that evade vaccination, but that is no reason to fear such a drastic reduction in its life expectancy. All vets will tell you that they see more and more very old cats, and these seniors (between eleven and fifteen years old) or geriatrics (over fifteen years old) often present with behavioral issues. I am always disappointed to find so little mention of behavioral issues among older cats in the abundant literature in English. Instead we have a catalogue of symptoms that are never grouped into the medical texts other than the general catchall term *cognitive dysfunction syndrome* (CDS).

This seems to suggest that there is only one form of behavioral illness once you get older. This is clearly not the case for human beings, so why would it be true for another animal with an equally complex behavioral repertoire? In fact, cats too experience diverse behavioral issues in old age, and let us bear in mind that aging in itself is not an illness.

The classification of illness within veterinary psychiatry recognizes at least four broad groups of behavioral issues that can feature in old age: emotional problems such as emotional dysregulation; thymic problems (touching on the animal's mood) such as involutional depression; purely cognitive problems such as confusion syndrome; and complex problems in which all three might be mixed together, such as hyper-aggressiveness in old cats.

Just as there are many forms of well-being, so it seems logical that there is no single behavioral disorder in advanced age. The distinction is not merely rhetorical. These different illnesses require different treatments and different therapies.

Léon: Lost in Translation

Let us begin with confusion syndrome, which in our use of the term is much less broad than the well-known CDS. Psychiatric vets make this diagnosis when we encounter pure cognitive issues in a cat without any elements of emotion or mood.

Léon suddenly became unclean at the age of fifteen. He was just as affectionate as ever, marked his territory by rubbing his cheek, and didn't seem to have changed a great deal. He wasn't leaping onto the furniture as much, he spent more time sleeping, and then, having been a model of cleanliness, started doing his business in strange places. His owners would often find him looking a little confused, a little harassed, lost on his way to the utility room, where his litter box had always been kept.

If, as was the case with Léon, there are a host of cognitive symptoms—loss of basic learning, disorientation, aimless wandering, confusion without any emotional cause—then there is a high chance of the cause being confusion syndrome, a feline illness analogous to Alzheimer's. Some important studies have shown that, as with humans and dogs,[21] a cat's brain can suffer a similar degeneration with amyloid over-load.[22] Just as there is currently no effective medical treat-ment for Alzheimer's, neither is there anything for cats (or dogs). Some potential treatments for Alzheimer's initially raised hopes, but these were soon dashed.

Knowing that there is no cure does not prevent us from treating a feline patient by helping to improve mental capacity and especially by rearranging their territory in order to adapt it to their changed needs. More litter boxes in more accessi-ble spots, comfortable sleeping places, and, also within easy reach, more gentle and predictable contact: all of this will help the affected cat to live longer and in greater comfort. In the case of Léon, the reorganization of his space and put-ting a litter box in a more accessible place made him clean again. Providing a few simple games and explaining the dis-ease helps the family to be there for the cat, accompanying it toward its final resting place, unhurriedly, enabling them to enjoy more precious months of life together.

THE INTERPRETATION OF CATS

Unhappy Harry

Harry had always been a nice cat, perhaps too nice—rather inhibited at least. A magnificent Burmese, he was brought to me when he was sixteen years old, because all of a sudden he was having terribly disrupted nights.

Harry would wander around the house meowing in a heartrending way: you only need to hear it once in your life to understand how unbearable this can be for humans, especially when they are attached to the cat. Harry, who seemed lost in his own home, was experiencing an inversion of his circadian rhythm (cats were originally nocturnal creatures, but on contact with humans they learned the rhythm of their owners and adapted to it) and above all seemed afraid, petrified in a space that was his and that he had known all his life. Add to this the loss of interest in daily activities (sometimes even including food) and a return to infantile behaviors (like chewing toys), and you will have a pretty good idea of the involutional depression of this old cat. When the distressed owner comes to the vet with this problem, there is a risk—less than it was but still there—that sedatives will be prescribed, frequently drugs that are tranquilizers and which depress the nervous system. They do not improve the symptoms; on the contrary, they can aggravate the animal's condition and make it more confused, or even aggressive, which in the vast majority of cases leads to it being put down.

As we saw earlier, the basis of a cat's mental well-being is its territory. Having to adapt to a less than optimal living space can trigger a permanent and inhibited anxious state that can become chronic depression, possibly complicated by thymic involution or regression to an earlier developmental stage. It is a serious situation, but there are solutions. Once we had checked that Harry was functioning well physically—his kidneys as well as his thyroid (old cats are very prone to hyperthyroidism)—we treated him with a brain-protecting psychotropic, to counter neuronal apoptosis (the death of neurons in the brain). We asked his humans to help make his life easier, simplifying his environment, making things more accessible and his routine more predictable, and everyone managed to find some peace.

The next recurrence, a little less than fifteen months later, which was foreseeable, proved resistant to treatment, and the decision was made not to allow his suffering to continue. Sometimes people say: "Is it worth it for a few extra months?" But who would turn their nose up at a few extra months of harmonious life? Harry's owners were delighted to rediscover the cat they knew and loved and to be able to continue to interact with him as before. They understood the situation—and were forewarned—and the extra months they gained were savored and helped them to prepare for the inevitable.

In behavioral medicine as in medicine generally, the aim is not always to find a cure, and maintaining a state of well-being is not always possible. So vets concentrate instead on quality of life. We are the guardians of the relationship between cats and their human companions.

The End of Life

Léon and Harry's afflictions are common in our pet cats. Such disorders in cats also act as a mirror, reflecting back our own questions about the type of old age we want for ourselves. Some people and animals as they grow older make us feel we want to age like them, while others reflect a terrible image of ongoing degradation that we want neither for ourselves nor for the animals who are dear to us. The most harrowing feeling is that of having no choice, being forced to grow old at whatever cost or having to keep our pet animals alive to the bitter end. I think we should all reflect together on this aspect of life. There are no easy answers, and there is probably no answer we will all agree upon, but the question is this: How can we cultivate both choice and dignity?

One should perhaps be surprised that there is no equivalent of an old people's home for aged animals, given that veterinary medicine explores the same disciplinary areas as human medicine. There is a rather obvious "Gordian" answer to this: when life becomes unbearable for pets, there is always the option of euthanasia. Some people will say that it is not the animal that makes the decision, and it's a valid point, but unless we question the right to have pets at all (and I think some animal rights extremists are not far off from that), we need to accept the idea that humans make all the significant decisions (sex, reproduction, food, shelter) on behalf of their animal companions. It seems contradictory to be angry at the irresponsibility of those who abandon their pets while,

at the same time, reproaching those who handle the important decisions in their pets' lives. It's a case of "You become
responsible, forever, for what you have tamed."[23] But is there
a limit to this? And, if so, who decides?

Once again, cats have become, despite themselves, the subject of a controversy concerning therapy and the limits of care.

Point Break: The Extreme Limit

In May 2019, Sushi, a three-year-old house cat, and Tara, a
small female Chartreux of the same age, made headlines. They
were the first cats in France to receive kidney transplants for
therapeutic reasons. This raised a few eyebrows: while some
people were amazed at the technical achievement it represented, others criticized an operation that they considered
unnecessary and over-the-top. Some posed the question: How
far is too far? Cats once again had made an impact and upset
conventional ways of thinking. Organ transplants, hitherto
the preserve of human beings, made available for house cats?

I confess I was surprised by all the outcry: veterinary medicine is not a drain on the public purse. There is no social
security, no state contribution: it should have remained a
private matter. But the furor in the press and the buzz on
social media brewed up a storm, and suddenly it all kicked
off. Praised by some, damned by others, the vets and the surgeon who achieved this milestone were subjected to a media
pile-on. I am on the executive council of the body that over-
sees the further education of general-practice vets in France,

the AFVAC.[24] When this all blew up, we were asked to form a small working group to consider the matter and formulate an official position for our profession. Two colleagues, both brilliant oncologists in internal medicine, and I had long discussions before publishing an article on the subject.[25]

It was a fascinating process, much less obvious than I might have thought at first, and fell into the category of "What are we getting ourselves into here?" This work on the limits of care took us into the vast field of medical ethics. This is still a new conceptual inquiry in veterinary medicine. Let us look at four pillars of medical ethics—autonomy, justice or equality, doing good, and doing no harm—and you will see why applying it to our profession is a complicated business.

The Principle of Autonomy

One of the principles that is becoming more and more respected in the field of human medicine is that of autonomy or freedom of choice: the patient should be able to decide if they want a given type of treatment or not. I am thinking here of certain anticancer treatments with low success rates that are offered to patients who have already suffered a great deal and who might opt not to have recourse to this last chance. We might also discuss this in terms of vaccines for certain diseases in which freedom of choice could have a wider impact and medical and government bodies decide that vaccination should be mandatory in order not to pose a risk to society as a whole.

In any case, this principle has enabled me to frame my approach in more precise terms: our pets cannot be autonomous; by definition, they are heteronomous—that is, all the decisions concerning their care are made by someone else, whether that is the person of attachment, the manager of a pet charity, or, ultimately, the vet. The best we can do is to ask the animal for its opinion, through observation and follow-up checking for signs of discomfort or, on the contrary, of pleasure, balancing our scientific knowledge with the importance of the relationship. In the article I wrote with my colleagues, we cited a case that one of my coauthors, Claire Beaudu-Lange, had experienced: Denzo, a small Bulldog, whose life expectancy after a diagnosis of advanced lymphoma T-cell was around three months according to scientific data. After discussions with his owners and because the little dog displayed a clear zest for life, treatment was undertaken, but Denzo died. Three months after treatment, and three days before his demise, he was still playing with his favorite stuffed toy.

To return to the kidney transplants, neither of the two cats could express its consent or its wishes, and the total absence of autonomy on the part of the donor is undoubtedly the issue that presents the thorniest problem to resolve. In human medicine, consent is sought at every stage and has to be stated explicitly. But for us vets, how do we resolve the moral issue of mutilating one animal for the benefit of another? A partial answer to this came from the United States, where anything that is not explicitly banned is permitted. With hindsight we are now able to state that cats who have had a kidney removed have encountered few complications and little loss of life expectancy. But that in itself is not sufficient justification for subjecting them to mutilation of this kind.

After some groping around in the dark, a new rule was brought in for all countries practicing transplants in cats. The donor must be a rescue cat, and clients who ask for an organ donation for their cat must commit to adopting the donor and offering it the same quality of life. This is still far short of autonomy, but at least there is a secondary benefit.

The Principle of Equality

This involves offering the same chances to each individual suffering from the same illness. No doubt in France, in human medicine, we try to respect this, but it would be unrealistic not to recognize that there is already (at least) a two-tier medical system, and if we look at the situation in the United States, this pillar of medical ethics is not in force at all.

To return to veterinary medicine, the average cost of a transplant is around €6,000, which is out of reach for many people, though we know some clients would not think twice about paying this money. In view of the importance that pets have for us, I am convinced that we will not be able to bring together ethics, the health of our cats, and our technical know-how until we make health insurance compulsory, a sort of private social security for animals. That would avoid all those heartrending cases where care has to end because of a lack of the means to pay for it. Vets, who have always been at the forefront of this fight but don't publicize it well enough, have recently relaunched an idea that germinated in my neck of the woods thirty years ago. Vétérinaires Pour Tous (Vets for All) is an organization that takes care of the animals of the most underprivileged people and makes up for the deficiencies or difficulties of certain owners. It is already a terrific initiative, but imagine if we had real solidarity among all pet owners. If dogs and cats were all insured, that would allow us to lower premiums and, by skimming the cream off a tiny part of the insurance costs, we could create a sustainable solidarity fund that would provide healthcare access for all.

We are never keen on additional financial obligations, but, to take one example, we accept it when it comes to our cars. I believe our pets are much more valuable to us. I would be happy in my final years in practice to contribute to setting up such a system, which would mean that never again would we be forced to refuse care. That first kidney transplant did not cost €6,000: the surgeon did it voluntarily for the sake of veterinary science and was excited at the prospect of saving a life "whatever it took," but in current practice there is no doubt that, without compulsory insurance—with a ceiling— this type of operation would be limited to cats whose owners were sufficiently well-off to pay for it.[26]

The Principles of Doing Good and Doing No Harm

Medicine should be of benefit to the patient; at the very least it should do no harm. In the case of the kidney transplant, the principle of doing good worked for the receiver, though it was far from evident for the donor. Now that we have the promise of an improvement in quality of life through adoption following the procedure, that is open to discussion, and everyone will have to form their own opinion.

What about sterilization? We have already aired the philosophical discussion of well-being linked to the decision to allow your cat access to its sexuality, but if we look at just the surgical procedure, does it fit in with the principle of doing good?

Some refer to this as an act of mutilation, and this offends many of my colleagues, who remain persuaded that by performing this operation they are doing good and resent being censured. I can only reiterate the point that it depends on the reasons for sterilization. In the case of population management, it is in fact counterproductive: for example, for this to work, it would be necessary to ensure that you have neutered all the male cats in the area; if you missed one, he could inseminate many females. From an individual and prophylactic point of view, neutering increases life expectancy by protecting against accidents and infection: it can be justified on medical grounds, even though such considerations also apply to humans but do not lead to the same conclusion. "Get neutered for a happy life" is not a common human motto. Vets are dedicated to animal health but do not lose sight of human health, and in a wider sense the environment. This can lead to ethical impasses that each must resolve according to their own conscience, in the absence of explicit rules and with changing social attitudes increasingly ready to call into question things that were previously regarded as self-evident.

This has allowed us to highlight the tensions that run through our society and drag our profession into an ethical debate. It is important to teach these notions of medical ethics; and that's what I and my colleagues at Toulouse University decided to do in our degree course in veterinary psychiatry. The vast majority of us practice an ethics of care. It is a pragmatic position, centered on the patient—in the strict sense of one who suffers—that allows us to take account not only of the animal but also of the relationship between it and the humans who accompany it.

Everything Went Well

To complete this roundup of complicated, and possibly insoluble, questions on later-life issues that our cats present us with, we must mention the debate on euthanasia. It overlaps the previous question on the limits of care. Most cats are not worth much in monetary terms. In fact, of the 700,000 cats acquired in France each year (the figures are quite difficult to assess exactly), only 50,000 have a pedigree and are pure breeds. These have a market value and are sometimes bought for several thousand euros. The rest are known as house cats or European cats, and are sold for a few hundred euros or less, or sometimes simply given away.

When medical care starts to rack up substantial fees, some people will ask themselves: Do I want to invest so much money in a cat that cost me nothing? In my experience, for most owners the two things bear no relation. Take the case of Luka: after a few days of shared existence, even though he had no monetary value, the humans who had taken him under their wing were ready to make a heavy investment—of time, of money, of suffering if needed—to preserve the relationship. Nevertheless, for others, the reality of their financial situation limits the amount of care they can provide. It is, I believe, also one of the reasons for the disenchantment of a certain number of young vets who leave college full of hope and ambition, used to working with the best technology, only to hit a wall of humdrum reality and client poverty. They will sometimes regard as pettiness or lack of attachment what is in fact just a limit for an owner who has to decide between caring for their cat and feeding their family. This creates a distortion, the feeling of a gulf between the professional ideal and reality that leads 25 percent of our students to abandon their practice within the first four years following their degree. And I am sure that this encounter with euthanasia is a big part of this disillusionment.

An important power vets have that is not shared by doctors is being able to decide, in agreement with those closest to the animal, to put an end to its days. Habitually having to present this option for consideration may help to explain, much more than access to drugs that will bring an end without suffering, the very high rates of suicide in our profession. A recent article comparing suicide rates of doctors and vets with those of the wider population pointed out that, while coming into contact with sickness and death was common to all the medical professions, the repeated stress involved in carrying out euthanasia, the decision-making as much as the act itself, was an aggravating factor for vets.[27] This partly explains a suicide rate four times higher than that of the general population. Today the ability to perform euthanasia can be even more of a poisoned chalice when vets run a greater risk of being challenged for carrying it out unless they can prove that they did so only after exhausting all other options.

Cats again bear particular witness to this: although they share with dogs and other animals the possibility of being put down when they are old or sick, it is only this species that faces the question of euthanasia for unwanted litters. Vets are all in agreement that it would be much better to prevent that through birth control, but once the kittens are there, usually in the springtime, what do you do? This frequently creates discussions among different members of the veterinary clinic, between those who are wholeheartedly opposed and those who are resigned to it for pragmatic reasons. Whatever the case, it is never an easy decision, and when vets do make it, it is to prevent it being done badly through drowning or asphyxiation in ether. Certain vets may refuse to do it, and that is their right. Even in the face of an administrative requisition, they might assert the right to refuse to participate in something that goes against their values. For us, euthanasia is and should remain a last therapeutic resort, when there is nothing else that can be done to prevent physical pain or mental suffering. It is a demanding privilege connected to the essential lack of self-determination of our domestic animals, of which cats are the prime examples, trapped between their image as cherished pets and being regarded as unwanted pests, as they are still considered by some local authorities, halfway between life at the heart of our homes and a semiferal existence in the wild.

At Cat College

Cats today have won the image battle. They are social media heroes. Their triumph tells us a lot about changes in our society and our relationship to education and hierarchy.

– Punishment Not Allowed

I'll say it again, one last time: all physical punishment of cats is forbidden. It never works and only creates the risk of a heightened sensitivity that can damage the relationship between a cat and its owner forever. For centuries, educating domestic animals was seen as a series of punishments and interdictions. While this does seem to work, unfortunately, in social species that are dependent on the relationship with their human owners, cats are intrinsically, essentially resistant to it.

Little by little, things have changed for everyone, and positive education is now the touchstone. Cats have gone along with this development. Nowadays you will find videos of cats doing parkour, high-fiving with their humans—in short, happy to learn and interact so long as they are respected and encouraged.

They teach us, then, that the best methods of education rely on collaborating with and engaging students. If that seems self-evident to you, don't forget that while it might be true here and now, it is not the case in the vast majority of the world.

– A Collaborative Culture

Our societies have long been based on hierarchy; the dog might act as a model of this. This is becoming less and less the case. Notions of authority and respect for elders have gone out of fashion, to be gradually replaced by a more horizontal and collaborative culture. The poster children for this development might be cats, as this is reminiscent of how groups of females can band together to share the care of kittens. Look around and you will see more and more examples of groups that operate without leaders, based on the sharing of tasks and a common objective. In dogs and in humans, when the hierarchy is clear, it can be comforting and provide the basis for building societies, but too often it can become anxiety-inducing and prevent self-realization. For cats, either the relationship is good and allows a communal life or it isn't, which leads to rupture. That is how project-based groups work: relationships are built around the common objective.

It is no surprise, then, that as longtime opponents of punishment and refuseniks of hierarchy, cats have become the representatives of this twenty-first-century style of doing things.

– The Body as Sacrosanct

The topic of sexual abuse, both past and present, is now more out in the open and has led to a different concept of the body as sacrosanct. Nowadays, before touching another person's body, you may do so only with their explicit permission. As we saw in the case of Isis, this also applies to a large degree to cats. Without comparing the traumatic experiences of people who have been abused with the desire of certain cats not to be touched, it is worth noting that here too our feline friend has been thrust into the role of spokesperson for a major cause. However, we must beware of exaggerating: some people are starting to claim that dogs don't like to be stroked, which seems very over-the-top to me. While it's true that some dogs don't like to be stroked and others don't like being stroked in a particular way, we should not draw general conclusions from that.

Some cats, even if not the majority, love physical contact and seek it out. Cats also tell us: be respectful of the other's body and open to everyone's uniqueness.

– Purr Therapy

They sometimes communicate this by purring, and this is still an enigma: a number of theories about these vibrations of the muscles of the larynx or the diaphragm have been advanced and subsequently disproved.

More importantly, there is the common misconception that purring is exclusively a sign of pleasure. But cats who are suffering, even dying, or giving birth, have been known to purr, and of course these situations involve pain or discomfort. One currently fashionable theory suggests that purring may have a healing role.[28] It occurs on a frequency between 25 and 50 Hz, which is the range of frequency that aids bone growth or scarring. Purring is a comforting message that the cat may address to itself in an unpleasant situation or to other partners with whom it is in harmony. It occurs first of all, naturally enough, between a mother and her kittens: the little ones are able to purr from as early as two days old, and the mothers do it during the birth and at feeding time.

Continue to make the most of it when your cat offers it to you: the peace that you feel when your cat purrs on your lap, or curled up next to you, is the soundtrack of your mutual trust.

– Personal Relations

This is the final lesson that we may take from our cats. While doing research for this book, I read a number of articles that spoke about social relations between cats or between cats and humans. This seemed to me to give a false impression: if we crossed out the word "social" every time it appeared, we might get closer to properly understanding cats. Their relationships are not social, or global, or automatic. Our domestic felines are experts in constructed relationships that require attention: they are fragile and reversible.

Cats don't love us because we are their "masters" and they laugh at the idea that we are their "owners." The fact that they belong to the same group, or are obliged to live in the same place, as us does not guarantee that a relationship will be established. But if you patiently build a connection with your cat, especially if the cat is sociable, with a natural tendency to want contact, to cultivate trust, and share moments of play and serenity, that provides the basis for establishing a real friendship.

* * *

In this brief review of the lessons that cats teach us, I have been assessing how many of my intuitions over the last twenty years have proved correct. The cat is iconic of our times because it represents values that are typically seen as feminine, qualities that our modern societies are assimilating more and more. Over the course of my adult life, I have seen the world—the Western world, at least—undergo a transition from a structure that might be defined as canine, coded masculine, hierarchical and vertical, whose dominant values are virility, even aggression and power, to a structure that is coded feminine, collaborative and horizontally structured, with values centered on quality of life, an emphasis on one's own space, and relationships, which comes close to a feline way of seeing things.

As I thought through these issues, I recalled a children's story by Rudyard Kipling about how, at a time when all animals were wild, domestication took place though the efforts of the first women, and how cats made a pact with them and obtained the right to come into the house, to be warm and well fed in exchange for keeping the children happy, making them laugh, and hunting mice. But, as cats wanted to keep their independence, they didn't sign a pact with men, who chase them from the house, or with dogs, "man's best friends," who run after them.[29] What is extraordinary is that Kipling wrote this story right at the beginning of the twentieth century, well before scientific discoveries showed us that domestication, or rather the connection between dogs and humans, probably occurred when they frequented the same living space (sympatry) and when female humans and female dogs observed how each other raised their young. Domestication of cats came much later and remains much more unstable.[30] What is even more striking is the evocation of this relationship between women and cats, which did not exclude all men (Kipling claimed that "three proper Men out of five will always throw things at a Cat whenever they meet him"), but which sealed a special alliance.

Together

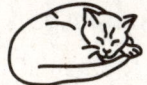

I've wanted to write this book for many years, and it has taken a long time to bring it to fruition. As well as recounting their stories, I spend most of my life caring for cats and teaching what is in my eyes the hugely important discipline of veterinary psychiatry. My hope is that I have responded to the request made by Prima in my dream to open up access to an understanding of cats, to give an insight into what it is like to be one, in order to help improve their quality of life.

As you will have grasped, this book is also an appeal to make up for the delay, to not abandon cats to their mental suffering. The 15 percent of cats undergoing medical consultation for behavioral issues are proof that we have not paid them enough attention, that we view them from a skewed perspective that prevents us from seeing them as they truly are and does them harm. Today, we are much better at diagnosing and treating feline behavioral issues, and even when they flirt with madness, we can still help them.

Cats are social media stars, sometimes adulated for the wrong reasons, often mistreated out of ignorance, and our enthusiasm must walk the path of knowledge. Throughout this book, I have tried to show the ways in which cats make us more empathetic. Doing the work involved opens the doors to a rich and complex world and can also allow us to discover the causes of certain illnesses and remedy them.

Cats also teach us about respect: observing the way they handle their bodies and their relationships forces us to step outside our human way of thinking if we wish to build a bridge between them and us. They are wonderful tightrope walkers, both physically and mentally, but their dual nature also exposes them to disorders that can produce suffering. All of this should not make us forget what is most important: the miracle of our interaction with them, the grace of their friendship, and the pleasure it gives us, a pleasure that can be . . . well, mad.

Notes

1 — The Joker, or the Dual Nature of the Cat

1 See the chapter "Idefix" in my book *La Psychologie du chien: Stress, anxiété, agressivité* [The Psychology of Dogs: Stress, Anxiety, Aggression] (Paris: Odile Jacob, 2004), p. 17.

2 See WSAVA (World Small Animal Veterinary Association), FECAVA (Federation of European Companion Animal Veterinary Associations), and AFVAC (Association française des vétérinaires pour animaux de compagnie).

3 M. E. Seligman and S. F. Maier, "Failure to escape traumatic shock," *Journal of Experimental Psychology*, 74 (1967), pp. 1–9.

4 B. Morizot, *Manières d'être vivant* [Ways of Being Alive] (Arles: Actes Sud, "Mondes sauvages," 2020).

5 U. Ferlier, "Campagne, ville ou environnement clos: quelle est l'influence du milieu de vie sur le répertoire comportemental du chat, à l'intérieur, chez ses propriétaires?" [Countryside, town, or enclosed space: what is the influence of the living environment on the behavioral repertoire of the cat, indoors, with its owners?], dissertation for a degree in behavioral veterinary medicine, University of Toulouse, October 2008.

2 — Territorial Problems

1 B. Werber, *Sa majesté des chats* [Her Majesty the Cat] (Paris: Albin Michel, 2019).

2 https://www.express.co.uk/news/weird/544409/Grumpy-Cat-worth -morethan-Hollywood-stars.

3 C. K. Kramer, S. Mehmood, and R. S. Suen, "Dog ownership and survival: a systematic review and meta-analysis," *Circulation: Cardiovascular Quality and Outcomes*, 12:10 (2019), e005554.

4 R. L. Zasloff, "Measuring attachment to companion animals: a dog is not a cat is not a bird," *Applied Animal Behaviour Science*, 47:1–2 (1996), pp. 43–8.

5 V. Despret, *Habiter en oiseau* [Live as a Bird] (Arles: Actes Sud, "Mondes sauvages," 2019).

6 A. Virring, R. Lambek, P. H. Thomsen, L. R. Moller, and P. J. Jennum, "Disturbed sleep in attention-deficit hyperactivity disorder (ADHD) is not a question of psychiatric comorbidity or ADHD presentation," *Journal of Sleep Research*, 25:3 (2016), pp. 333–40.

7 For example, P. Leyhausen, *Cat Behavior: The Predatory and Social Behavior of Domestic and Wild Cats* (New York: Garland STPM Press, 1979).

8 V. Villeneuve-Beugnet and F. Beugnet, "Field assessment of cats' litter box substrate preferences," *Journal of Veterinary Behavior*, 25 (2018), pp. 65–70.

9 J. J. Ellis, R. T. S. McGowan, and F. Martin, "Does previous use affect litter box appeal in multi-cat households?," *Behavioural Processes*, 141 (2017), pp. 284–90.

10 E. K. Grigg, L. Pick, and B. Nibblett, "Litter box preference in domestic cats: covered versus uncovered," *Journal of Feline Medicine and Surgery*, 15:4 (2013), pp. 280–84 (© ISFM and AAFP, 2012).

11 MNHN (National Museum of Natural History) and SFEPM research, http://www.chat-biodiversite.fr.

12 C. Béata, *Au risque d'aimer* [The Danger of Loving] (Paris: Odile Jacob, 2013).

13 L. Monti-Bloch, C. Jennings-White, and D. L. Berliner, "The human vomeronasal system: a review," *Annals of the New York Academy of Sciences*, 855 (1998), pp. 373–89.

3 — To Relate or Not to Relate

1 C. Béata and G. Muller (eds.), *Pathologie du comportement du chat* [Cat Behavioral Pathology] (Paris: Éditions AFVAC, 2016).

2 S. Schwartz, "Separation anxiety syndrome in dogs and cats," *Journal of the American Veterinary Medical Association*, 222 (2003), pp. 1526–32.

3 J.-D. Vigne et al., "Early taming of the cat in Cyprus," *Science*, 304: 5668 (2004), p. 259.

4 P. Pageat, *Pathologie du comportement du chien* [Dog Behavioral Pathology] (Paris: Éditions du Point Vétérinaire, 1994).

5 J. Hofmans, "Étude clinique sur chatons. Inhibition du chaton à 6 semaines et tempérament à 6 mois: qu'en est-il?" [Clinical study on kittens. Inhibition of the kitten at 6 weeks and temperament at 6 months: what is it?], dissertation for a degree in behavioral veterinary medicine, Toulouse University, 2021.

6 Constitution of the World Health Organization, 1946.

7 Vigne et al., "Early taming of the cat in Cyprus."

8 N. Russell, "The wild side of animal domestication," *Society and Animals*, 10:3 (2002), pp. 285–302.

9 AAFP (American Association of Feline Practitioners) and ISFM (International Society of Feline Medicine), "Feline environmental needs guidelines," *Journal of Feline Medicine and Surgery*, 15 (2013), pp. 219–30.

10 Simon's Cat, "Cat Man Do," https://www.youtube.com/watch?v=V8os2v7ZuJs.

11 Béata, *Au risque d'aimer*.

12 Ibid.

13 S. Crowell-Davis, "Understanding cats," *Compendium: Continuing Education for Veterinarians*, 29:4 (2007), pp. 241–3.

4 — One Flew Over the Cat's Nest

1 M. Kreutzer, *Folies animales* [Animal Madness] (Paris: Le Pommier, 2020).

2 H. Ey and A. Brion, *Psychiatrie animale* [Animal Psychiatry] (Paris: Desclée de Brouwer, 1964).

3 Béata, *Au risque d'aimer*.

4 *Blackfish*, film by Gabriela Cowperthwaite, 2013.

5 B. Garner et al., "Pituitary volume predicts future transition to psychosis in individuals at ultra-high risk of developing psychosis," *Biological Psychiatry*, 58 (2005), pp. 417–23; E. S. Brown, A. J. Rush, and B. S. McEwen, "Hippocampal remodeling and damage by

corticosteroids: implications for mood disorders," *Neuropsychophar-macology*, 21 (1999), pp. 474–84.

6 P. Watzlawick and Giorgio Nardone, *Stratégie de la thérapie brève* [Brief Strategic Therapy] (Paris: Seuil, 1998).

7 LOOF: L'Abyssin, https://www.loof.asso.fr/races/desc_race.php?id _race=1.

8 J.-P. Sastre and M. Jouvet, "The oneiric behavior of the cat," *Physiology & Behavior*, 22:5 (1979), pp. 979–89.

9 J. Ferguson and W. C. Dement, "The effect of variations in total sleep time on the occurrence of rapid eye movement sleep in cats," *Electro-encephalography and Clinical Neurophysiology*, 22 (1967), pp. 2–10; M. A. Carskadon and W. C. Dement, "Monitoring and staging human sleep," in M. H. Kryger, T. Roth, and W. C. Dement (eds.), *Principles and Practice of Sleep Medicine*, 5th edition (St. Louis, MO: Elsevier Saunders, 2011), pp. 16–26.

10 A. Lauveng, *Demain j'étais folle: un voyage en schizophrénie* [Tomorrow I Was Mad: A Journey into Schizophrenia] (Paris: Autrement, 2019).

11 O. Jacqmot, "Comparison of several white matter tracts in feline and canine brain by using magnetic resonance diffusion tensor imaging," *Anatomical Record*, 300 (2017), pp. 1270–89.

12 L. Naccache, *Le Nouvel Inconscient: Freud, le Christophe Colomb des neurosciences* [The New Unconscious: Freud, the Christopher Colum-bus of Neuroscience] (Paris: Odile Jacob, 2006).

13 L. U. Sneddon, "Pain perception in fish: indicators and endpoints," *ILAR Journal*, 50:4 (2009), pp. 338–42.

14 J. L. Owens, M. Olsen, A. Fontaine, C. Kloth, A. Kershenbaum, and S. Waller, "Visual classification of feral cat *Felis silvestris catus* vocaliza-tions," *Current Zoology*, 63 (2017), pp. 331–39; C. Tavernier, S. Ahmed, K. A. Houpt, and S. C. Yeon, "Feline vocal communication," *Journal of Veterinary Science*, 21:1 (2020), e18.

15 G. G. Gallup, "Chimpanzees: self-recognition," *Science*, 167: 3914 (Jan-uary 2, 1970), pp. 86–7.

5 — A Symbol of Our Time

1 A. R. Damasio, *Descartes' Error: Emotion, Reason, and the Human Brain*, revised edition (London: Vintage, 2006).

2 E. S. Steigerwald, M. Sarter, P. March, and M. Podell, "Effects of feline immunodeficiency virus on cognition and behavioral function in cats," *Journal of Acquired Immune Deficiency Syndromes and Human Retrovirology*, 20:5 (1990), pp. 411–19.

3 J.-P. Beaufils, "Modifications du comportement induites par le virus de l'imunodéficience féline (FIV) chez le chat" [Behavioral changes induced by feline immunodeficiency virus (FIV) in cats], dissertation for the degree in behavioral veterinary medicine, Toulouse University, 2001.

4 C. A. Buffington, D. J. Chew, and B. E. Woodworth, "Feline interstitial cystitis," *Journal of the American Veterinary Medical Association*, 215 (1999), pp. 682–7.

5 Ibid. and C. A. Buffington, J. L. Westropp, D. J. Chew, and R. R. Bolus, "Clinical evaluation of multimodal environmental modification (MEMO) in the management of cats with idiopathic cystitis," *Journal of Feline Medicine and Surgery*, 8:4 (2006), pp. 261–68.

6 C. A. Buffington and M. Bain, "Stress and feline health," *Veterinary Clinics of North America: Small Animal Practice*, 50:4 (2020), pp. 653–62.

7 C. A. Buffington, "Pandora syndrome in cats: diagnosis and treatment," *Today's Veterinary Practice*, Autumn 2018, pp. 31–40, https://todaysveterinarypractice.com/urology-renal-medicine/pandora-syndrome-in-cats/.

8 S. Denenberg (ed.), *Small Animal Veterinary Psychiatry* (Wallingford, England: CABI Publishing, 2020).

9 É. Zola, "Le paradis des chats" [Cat Paradise], in *Nouveaux contes à Ninon* [New Tales for Ninon], 1874.

10 Ferlier, "Campagne, ville ou environnement clos."

11 B. Vian, *L'Arrache-cœur* [Heartsnatcher] (Paris: Le Livre de Poche, 1953).

12 W. P. Stubbs and M. S. Bloomberg, "Implications of early neutering in the dog and cat," *Seminars in Veterinary Medicine and Surgery (Small Animal)*, 10:1 (1995), pp. 8–12.

13 C. V. Spain, J. M. Scarlett, and K. A. Houpt, "Long-term risks and benefits of early-age gonadectomy in cats," *Journal of the American Veterinary Medical Association*, 224 (2004), pp. 372–79.

14 M. A. Kutzler, "Possible relationship between long-term adverse health effects of gonad-removing surgical sterilization and luteinizing hormone in dogs," *Animals*, 10:4 (2020), p. 599.

15 Béata, *Au risque d'aimer*.

16 D. J. Mellor, "Positive animal welfare states and encouraging environment-focused and animal-to-animal interactive behaviours," *New Zealand Veterinary Journal*, 63:1 (2015), pp. 9–16.

17 Agence nationale de sécurité sanitaire de l'alimentation, de l'environnement et du travail (French National Agency for Health Security), 14, rue Pierre-et-Marie-Curie, 94701 Maisons-Alfort.

18 Béata, *Au risque d'aimer*.

19 T. Lodé, *La Guerre des sexes chez les animaux* [War of the Sexes in Animals] (Paris: Odile Jacob, 2007); *La Biodiversité amoureuse: sexe et évolution* [Biodiversity in Love: Sex and Evolution] (Paris: Odile Jacob, 2011); *Pourquoi les animaux trichent et se trompent: les infidélités de l'évolution* [Why Animals Cheat and Make Mistakes: The Infidelities of Evolution] (Paris: Odile Jacob, 2013); *Histoire naturelle du plaisir amoureux* [The Natural History of Sexual Pleasure] (Paris: Odile Jacob, 2021).

20 "Le chat d'exterieur est-il plus heureux que le chat d'interieur?" ["Is an outdoor cat happier than an indoor cat?"], on the Wamiz website, https://wamiz.com/chats/conseil/le-chat-doit-il-sortir-pour-etre-heureux-3459.html.

21 C. Béata, *La Psychologie du chien*, chapter 7, "Kim," p. 287.

22 Feline illness is even closer to the human variety: while there is no neurofibrillary degeneration, as in humans but never in dogs, hyperphosphorylated tau proteins may be present, as in humans, though not in dogs. D. A. Gunn-Moore, J. Mcvee, J. M. Bradshaw, G. R. Pearson, E. Head, and F. J. Gunn-Moore, "Ageing changes in cat brains demonstrated by beta-amyloid and AT8-immunoreactive phosphorylated tau deposits," *Journal of Feline Medicine and Surgery*, 8 (2006), pp. 234–42; E. Head, K. Moffat, P. Das, F. Sarsoza, W. W. Poon, G. Landsberg, C. W. Cotman, and M. P. Murphy, "Beta-amyloid deposition and tau phosphorylation in clinically characterized aged cats," *Neurobiology of Aging*, 26 (2005), pp. 749–63.

23 Antoine de Saint-Exupéry, *The Little Prince*, trans. T. V. F. Cuffe (London: Penguin, 1995), p. 72.

24 AFVAC: Association française des vétérinaires pour animaux de compagnie (French Association of Vets for Companion Animals), 40, rue de Berri, 75008 Paris.

25 C. Béata, C. Beaudu-Lange, and C. Muller, "Jusqu'où va-t-on dans les soins donnés à nos animaux de compagnie?" [How far should we go in caring for our pets?], *Revue vétérinaire clinique*, 56:4 (2021), pp. 157–69.

26 F. Mereo, "Greffe de rein sur un chat: 'Sauver une vie, quelle qu'elle soit, est gratifiant'" [Kidney transplant on a cat: "Saving a life, of any kind, is rewarding"], *Le Parisien*, 21 August 2019.

27 E. L. Fink-Miller and L. M. Nestler, "Suicide in physicians and veterinarians: risk factors and theories," *Current Opinion in Psychology*, 22 (2018), pp. 23–6.

28 E. von Muggenthaler, "The felid purr: a bio-mechanical healing mechanism," in *12th International Conference on Low Frequency Noise and Vibration and Its Control*, conference report published in Bristol, UK, September 18–20, 2006.

29 R. Kipling, "The cat that walked by himself," in *Just So Stories* (London: Macmillan, 1902), https://etc.usf.edu/lit2go/79/just-so-stories/1296/the-cat-that-walked-by-himself/.

30 M. Pionnier-Capitan, C. Bemilli, P. Bodu, G. Celerier, J.-G. Ferrie, P. Fosse, M. Garcia, and J.-D. Vigne, "New evidence for Upper Palaeolithic small domestic dogs in South-Western Europe," *Journal of Archaeological Science*, 38 (2011), pp. 2123–40.